SECRETS OF THE SEX MASTERS

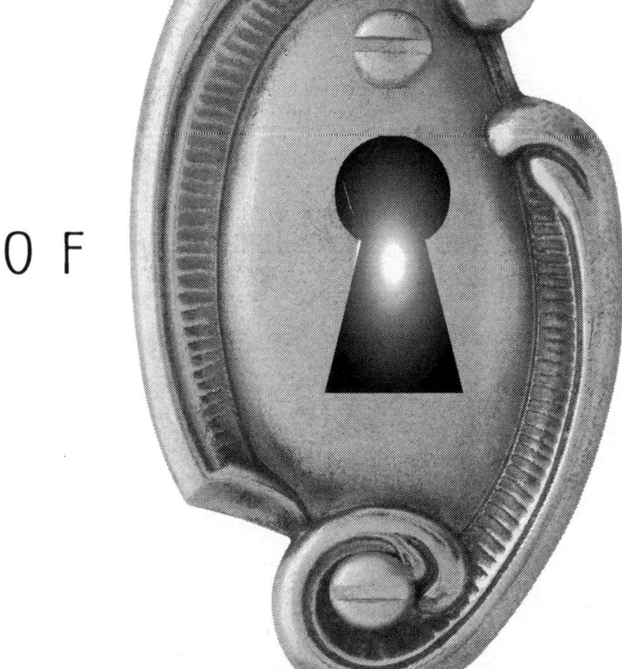

CO-WRITTEN & EDITED BY CARL FRANKEL

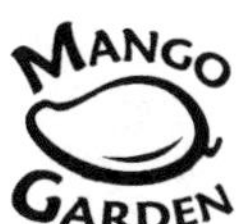

MANGO GARDEN PRESS · KINGSTON, NEW YORK

About Mango Garden Press and the Center for the Intimate Arts

Mango Garden Press is the publishing arm of Sheri Winston's Center for the Intimate Arts. The mission of Mango Garden Press and the Center for the Intimate Arts is to provide empowering, enlightening, entertaining erotic education for everyone.

We envision a world where sex is understood, honored and free from shame, where our bodies' ecstatic potential is explored and celebrated, and relationships are based on integrity, compassion and love.

Our products and services include:

In-person and online classes, workshops and presentations for lay people and professionals.

Individual and couples coaching and counseling (in-person and via phone/skype).

Books in digital and hard-copy format, which we publish via our imprint, Mango Garden Press. For more information, visit MangoGardenPress.com.

Articles, written blogs and video 'vlogs' by Sheri Winston and Carl Frankel. These can be found on our website as well in articles by Carl Frankel at YourTango.com.

For more information or to sign up for our newsletter, please visit us at IntimateArtsCenter.com.

Cover & Interior Design: Tilman Reitzle

Illustrations: Christopher King/Dreamstime (cover);
Sheri Winston (Chapters 1 and 16) ; Amy Noseworthy (Chapter 2)

Photo Credits: FlamingPumpkin/iStock (cover & title page)

Author Photo Identifier (back cover)—*clockwise, from bottom left*:
Patricia Taylor, Karen B.K. Chan, Carl Frankel, Jessica O'Reilly, Reid Mihalko, Sheri Winston, Charles Muir, Caroline Muir, Joseph Kramer, Eve Minax, Michael Winn, Jaeleen Bennis, Charlie Glickman, Megan Andelloux, Carlyle Jansen, Tallulah Sulis, Ernest Greene, Nadine Thornhill, Nina Hartley, Jon Pressick

ISBN 978-0-9898138-4-6
Library of Congress #: 2014917112

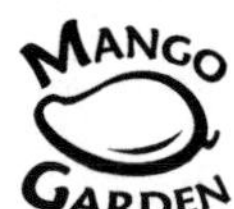

Mango Garden Press
PO Box 3184
Kingston, NY 12402
www.MangoGardenPress.com

Printed on Forest Stewardship Council-certified, 30% post-consumer recycled paper.

Contents

We hold these truths to be self-evident, that all men are created equal, that they are endowed by their Creator with certain unalienable Rights, that among these are Life, Liberty and the pursuit of Erotic Happiness.

—The U.S. Declaration of Independence
[tweaked]

Acknowledgments

NO BOOK IS TRULY A SOLO PROJECT. Authors are influenced by friends, lovers, family, other writers and much more. This is true for bad writing, it's true for good writing, and it's especially true for this work, which would not exist but for the contributions of the sex masters of the title.

So: My heartfelt thanks to the 'sexperts' who contributed their time, knowledge and talents to this project: Carlyle Jansen, Caroline Muir, Charles Muir, Charlie Glickman, Ernest Greene, Eve Minax, Jaeleen Bennis, Jessica O'Reilly, Jon Pressick, Joseph Kramer, Karen B.K. Chan, Megan Andelloux, Michael Winn, Nadine Thornhill, Nina Hartley, Patti Taylor, Reid Mihalko, Sheri Winston and Tallulah Sulis. I am grateful to you both for appreciating the project's potential and for your collegial collaboration.

A special shout-out goes to my life and business partner Sheri Winston, who also contributed a chapter. As I write this, we've been together going on nine years. Through and alongside her, I have come to know an extraordinary community of people who are individually and collectively committed to creating a world with a healthy, responsible, celebratory attitude towards sex. These people are passionate about their vision; they are passionate about passion; and some of the best and most passionate contributed to this book.

Sheri, thank you for introducing me to this fun and fascinating world. Thank you for the many gifts you've given me. Thank you for your integrity, intelligence, companionship and support.

Thanks also to our colleagues Bryan Thomlison, Fatima Nasim and Cynthia S. for keeping our business humming while my head was down in this book.

Thank you, Val Vadeboncoeur, for your stellar proofing and copy-editing contributions. And thank you, Leilani Arenas, for being such a courteous, skilled and easy to work with transcriber.

Thank you, Tilman Reitzle. You are a book-design orisha. Sheri and I place offerings at your altar—and in your bank account—regularly.

* * *

When Sheri and I first got together, I was middle-aged. Which makes me middler-aged now. It's said that you can't teach an old dog new tricks, but I beg, woof woof, to differ. I've learned new tricks. Sex-master tricks.

Compiling and editing this book has been good for me. I hope it will be good for you, too.

Introduction

by Carl Frankel

WE ALL HAVE DIFFERENT APTITUDES. Joe is great at math but terrible at reading social signals. Carl's smooth in the salon, but present him with a mechanical challenge and he becomes a small domestic animal confronting a Rubik's Cube.

Some people—the lucky ones—are gifted at sex. *Really* gifted at sex.

These are the sex masters of this book's title. They're clear channels about matters erotic.

For many of us, sex is as confusing as it is compelling. For this we can thank, if that's the word for it, a triumvirate of factors: the hugely powerful nature of the sex drive, the urgent need to control it so as not to harm ourselves and others—kind of like managing a hurricane—and, last but not least, our culture's ignorant, misguided and often sex-negative views about the entire territory. Put these together—the power of lust, our need to channel it, and our culture's wildly mixed messages—and it's no wonder that a great many of us don't know which end is up when it comes to that wild energy running through our loins.

The sex masters of these pages missed out on all that confusion, or got past it somehow. They see sex for what it really is, beyond and behind all the trappings it comes bedecked in. And what do they see, exactly?

A magnificent gift.

An unparalleled way to connect.

A source of amazing pleasure.

And, on a parallel note, they see a human tragedy in all the sex-negativity that's out there.

They also know how good sex can be, which is a lot better than your average bear—or human—believes possible. They understand that there's sex the way it's usually done, and there's sex the mind-blowing, boundary-busting, better-than-you-could-ever-imagine way. And they see both kinds of sex—but especially the second kind of sex, the 'super-sex' kind of sex, the sex that so many people don't know about—as our erotic birthright.

The usual sexual scenario features limited foreplay, a single ejaculatory orgasm by the man and an orgasm or two by the woman . . . sometimes, maybe.

(This is, of course, the heterosexual version. Adjust as appropriate for gay.)

And then there's the insanely ecstatic alternative—leisurely foreplay that can lead to full-body, non-ejaculatory 'dry' orgasms for the man and massive 'megasms' for the woman that continue for hours and hours.

To do Shakespeare a gross disservice: *There are more things in heaven and earth, Horatio, than are dreamt of in your pornography.*

If this sounds over the top—the sex, not the wordplay—it's not. I've both witnessed and experienced these things and I'm not even a sex master. The difference between your usual sex and the amazing, transcendent sex that these sex masters teach and practice is like the difference between a country-club golf champion and a touring pro. Same sport, different league.

Are these people special? Yes—they have secret knowledge—and no—they're just folks. With the right attitude and information—all laid out in these pages—you can, as they say, have what they're having.

That's why I curated this project. So you could be a sex master, too.

Not Just Technical Guidance

When I launched *Secrets of the Sex Masters*, I assumed I'd be assembling a range of technical guidance on how to be a great lover. And I have. In these pages, you'll find chapters on Tantra (Charles Muir), male non-ejaculatory orgasm (Michael Winn), female expanded orgasm (Patti Taylor), energy sex (Reid Mihalko), female ejaculation (Tallulah Sulis), female genital anatomy and sexuality (Sheri Winston), oral sex (Carlyle Jansen) and anal sex (Jon Pressick). There is technical guidance a-plenty here.

But the book turned out to be more than that. Time and again, I found these 'sexperts' addressing the 'why' of sex along with the 'how to.' They kept stressing that sex isn't only about physical pleasure, it's also about *connecting.* Over a century ago, the novelist E.M. Forster had an improbably prescient epigram in his novel *Howard's End*: "Only connect." It's an attitude shared by the sex masters, with this addendum: "And a great way to connect is through (responsible) sex."

What I eventually came to think of as 'my' sex masters also spent an unexpected amount of time discussing our many emotional obstacles to connecting. By the time the book was done, I had a chapter on sex and shame (Charlie Glickman), one on (among other things) honoring our erotic fantasies (Megan Andelloux), and another on finding the lover within (Caroline Muir).

The importance of communication also kept cropping up. When I asked kink experts Nina Hartley and Ernest Greene to give me their list of most important things to be expert at, I expected answers like "honor limits" and "stay in character." Nope: Communication was head and shoulders above everything else.

Eventually I came to understand that these weren't just sex geeks with specialized knowledge I was interviewing. These were wise people who understand deep down that being the proverbial 'wonderful lover' isn't only about touch skills, erotic breathing and the like. It's also about . . . duh! . . . loving wonderfully. It's about bringing your heart and all the rest of you—mind, body, spirit—to your erotic encounters. It's about loving well and being full of wonder—about your partner, about the experience, about the Mystery—whether you're with a long-term partner, a friend with benefits, or someone you just met.

So: What you hold in your hands isn't only a sex book about how to be good in bed. It's also a wisdom book about how to be fully human.

And to be that way in the bedroom.

Fully human: Now, that's hot!

It turns out that one of the keys to being a great lover is to show up as you truly are. This makes exquisite sense if you give it a moment's thought: How can you connect with another person if you're not really there? And how can they connect with you? Masks don't connect and ghosts don't, either.

Sex, these clear channels and wise beings kept stressing, isn't only about physical ecstasy.

It's also about connecting.

The Story Behind This Book

It may be useful for me to share a few words about how I came to this project. I've been partnered with the award-winning sex teacher Sheri Winston since 2005. In 2009, I began collaborating with her in her business, The Center for the Intimate Arts. This was a new professional direction for me in the sense that I was neither a sex nor intimacy professional. Yet it was also a continuation of my old path because it involved entrepreneurship, writing and editing, my work for three decades, and because this was a social enterprise—business with a dual commitment to doing good and doing well—and this was my main area of expertise.

Over time, I came to know Sheri's colleagues, many of whom were also her friends. Inveterate entrepreneur that I am, it wasn't long before I'd dreamed up the Secrets of the Sex Masters concept. I now knew some of the best sexperts in the United States. Why not leverage their collected knowledge into a book that would help get their important sex-positive guidance out into the world? This project was totally in my wheelhouse and would be fun, too.

Eventually I started reaching out to some of the sex teachers I knew. Just about everyone I invited to participate liked both the concept and the collaborative nature of my proposed approach. I wasn't asking them simply to deliver a chapter to me: I'd work with them to make it happen, first by interviewing them and then by proactively using my writing and editing skills to help them transform the transcript into a chapter we were both proud of. This meant less work for them and, busy people that they are, they appreciated this.*

I knew many but not all the contributors when I launched this project. The retired porn actress and self-proclaimed 'sexecologist' Annie Sprinkle referred me to Eve Minax ('Eroticizing Safer Sex') and Jaeleen Bennis ('Bondassage'). A friend of Sheri's recommended the Taoist master Michael Winn. Contributor Carlyle Jansen introduced me to sex blogger and fellow Torontonian Jon Pressick ("Anal Sex").

One connection happened without the benefit of an introduction. I'd read somewhere that the famous porn actress Nina Hartley—one of the few porn 'stars' out there genuinely worthy of the name—was an 'out' submissive and took it upon myself to contact her and her husband, the dominant Ernest Greene, for the chapter on kink. They received my overture graciously and we had a great conversation.

Seventeen chapters, nineteen sex masters, a wealth of practical information and technical guidance, and a heaping helping of wisdom, too.

All for one purpose—so you, like the authors of these chapters, can become a clear channel about sex and fully claim your erotic birthright.

Enjoy!

*** In five of the seventeen chapters, I played an editing, not co-authoring, role.**

Essential Information

A celebrated author and Wholistic Sexuality educator, **SHERI WINSTON** CNM, RN, BSN, LMT *has been on a learning journey about sex for most of her life. In following her first calling as a midwife, she inadvertently discovered how to have better sex, easier orgasms and fabulous erotic relationships. Her personal experiences led to her to consciously study the full spectrum of human sexuality, including Western medicine, and sexology, holistic healing, ancient and contemporary sacred sexuality traditions . When she retired from attending births, her second calling was born—teaching men, women, singles, and partners about their sexuality—supporting them to give birth to their inherent erotic potential.*

Sheri is the author of the award-winning Women's Anatomy of Arousal: Secret Maps to Buried Pleasure,* *and* Succulent SexCraft: Your Hands-On Guide to Erotic Play and Practice. Women's Anatomy of Arousal *has been called "the most comprehensive, user-friendly, practical and uplifting book on women's sexuality I have ever read" by the educator and author Dr. Christiane Northrup.* Succulent SexCraft *has been garnering rave reviews and achieved #1 status among books about sex on Amazon. It's a visionary yet practical guide to becoming an erotic virtuoso and masterful lover.*

As the founder and executive director of the Center for the Intimate Arts, Sheri offers empowering entertaining erotic education, in-person and online. Sheri's classes are renowned for their integral perspective and broad range of knowledge, as well as their comfort, humor and transformational potential. They cover a wide range of sex-related topics, including orgasmic abundance, the anatomy of arousal, sexual techniques, erotic communication and relationship skills.

Sheri's unique and holistic teachings are informed by her fifteen years as a sexuality teacher on top of over two decades of practice as a certified nurse-midwife, gynecology practitioner, registered nurse, holistic healer, childbirth educator, doula, artist and massage therapist.

Sheri teaches her wide and varied curriculum of Intimate Arts and Wholistic Sexuality classes to the general public and also offers professional level trainings for other sexuality educators and health care providers. Sheri delights in inspiring folks of all kinds and ages to have a lot more pleasure, fun and fulfillment!

More info: IntimateArtsCenter.com.

***Winner, 2010 Book of the Year Award—American Association of Sex Educators, Counselors and Therapists (AASECT)**

CHAPTER ONE

The Dance of Anatomy and Energy

by Sheri Winston

ART BY SHERI WINSTON

IF YOU WANT TO GET TO THE LAND OF AMAZING EROTIC EXPERIENCES, it helps to have an accurate map. Maps, actually.

For starters, it helps to know your sexual equipment and that of your partners—what's there, how it works and how to get the most pleasure possible.

Given all the interest in sex now and throughout history, you'd think your average Joe and Josephina would be pretty sophisticated about the relevant anatomy. Not so. Many people don't even have the anatomy basics that you'll find in sex books and text books. But the challenge goes beyond that. Even the vast majority of people with basic knowledge don't have the whole picture. Our cultural maps of sexual parts are incomplete and sometimes just plain wrong. Strange but true: Despite contemporary science's amazing advances, we still don't have a comprehensive understanding of what's down there or how it's all connected.

Outer space isn't our only frontier. There's also our genitals.

We're also missing useful maps for understanding sexual energy—what it is, how it operates and the power of polarity. Many people are especially confused about sexual polarity. We can think of these polarities as 'giving and getting,' 'penetrating and receiving' or 'masculine and feminine.' (I'm referring here to energy, not plumbing.) When it comes to sexual energy, for most of us, one polarity is stronger than the other. An accurate map of sexual polarity enables us to be more skilled at navigating our own sexuality and our erotic connections.

I regret this lack of knowledge. The absence of accurate maps reduces people's capacity to give and receive pleasure and to understand and consciously play

*** Chapter 15 is also about sexual energy, but its focus is on how to play with erotic energy, not on sexual polarity. That's why aspects of sexual energy other than polarity aren't discussed here.**

with sexual polarity. The result: In the bedroom, most people are like airplane pilots who are flying their craft with limited or inaccurate instrumentation. They don't reach their full sexual potential or know how to help their partners achieve theirs.

In this chapter, I'll provide maps of genital anatomy and sexual energy polarity that will help you lift your bedroom sessions to new levels of bliss.

The Female Erectile Network

As you may already know, erectile tissue is what gives the penis its hallmark ability to go from small and soft to big and hard. But 'erectability' isn't only a property of penises. Here's an anatomical fact about female equipment most people find astonishing: *Women have as much erectile tissue as men.* Pound for pound and inch for inch, women have just as much of this wonderful, expandable, engorgeable equipment as men. The female erectile network is made up of a number of linked structures, all comprised of enlargeable, sweetly swelling, inflatable erectile tissue. Knowing where all this erectable equipment is located is a foundational map for owners and visitors.

Women have as much erectile tissue as men.

We'll start our tour of the *female erectile network* with the clitoris. Despite the common misconception that the clitoris is only the acorn-shaped nub, it actually has three parts. What is generally thought of as the clitoris is actually the *clitoral head* or *glans*. With 6,000-8,000 nerve endings, it's the jewel in the crown of the female pleasure system—the tip of the volcano, as it were. This is the largest concentration of nerve endings in the male or female body. Being such a super-sensitive spot means that the clitoral head can easily be over-stimulated. As with so many things, timing is crucial for playing with this special part. Generally speaking—genitally speaking, really—most women don't want direct clitoral stimulation until they're already at a high level of arousal. Also, after orgasm, many women have a period of hypersensitivity when direct stimulation is too much. Clitoral visitors, you need to check in and be aware that the clitoral head wants different things at different times.

The next part of the clitoris, the *clitoral shaft* (also known as the *body* or *corpus*), can be found under the hood, just above the head of the clitoris. This small pole is about the width of a chopstick or a pencil and is about one-half to one inch long. It rests in a slightly mobile tube. The clitoral shaft is wonderful to play with—it's made up of sensitive erectile tissue, but isn't as super-delicate as the head. It's also protected by the clitoral hood. This makes it a good target for stimulation when a woman is in medium-level arousal.

The paired *clitoral legs* are the third part of the clitoris. They branch from the base of the shaft like a wishbone and head south, running along the sides of the bony pubic arch. Only the top parts of the legs are palpable, and even they can usually be felt only at high arousal.

All three parts of the clitoris—the head, shaft and paired legs—are made up of erectile tissue. Just like a penis, the whole clitoris has the ability to become engorged, filling with blood and getting bigger, firmer and more sensitive.

But that's not all.

Under the outer labia, beneath a layer of muscle are two big wads of engorgeable erogenous tissue—the paired *vestibular bulbs*. Each is shaped like an upside-down comma, fat at the bottom, thin at the top. They bracket the vaginal orifice. When swollen, they help form the sides of the snug cuff that encircles the vaginal opening. In additional to adding pleasurable sensations directly, the top of each bulb connects to the shaft of the clitoris. When the bulbs are puffed, they transmit additional delightful stimulation to the sensitive clitoral system. The vestibular bulbs can be pleasured by rubbing the tissue under the outer labia. Once you know that they're there, you'll discover that they love broad diffuse strokes and firm rubbing. The bulbs are a great part of the female genitalia to play with first. When they're properly attended to, they puff up considerably and get the whole erectile network jumpstarted.

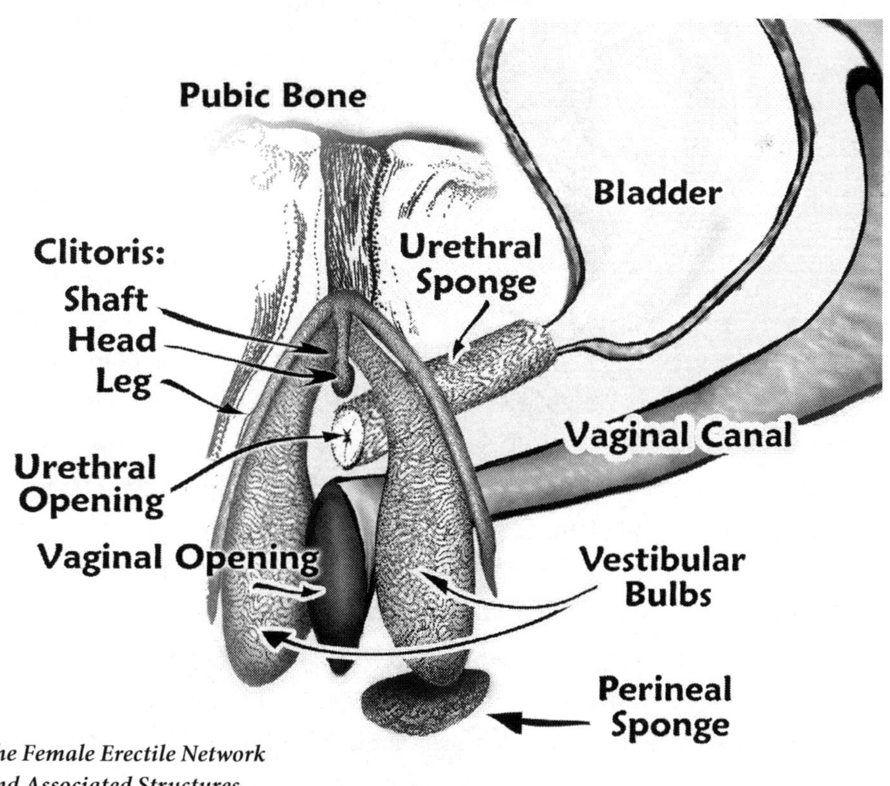

The Female Erectile Network and Associated Structures

And there's more.

Inside the female body are two more erectile structures. The urethral sponge (the bottom of which is commonly known as the G-spot) is a cylinder of erectile tissue that surrounds the tube of the urethra.* It lies just above and parallel to the roof of the vagina. The urethral sponge can be compared to a roll of paper towels. The urethra (the pee tube) is the cardboard cylinder and the surrounding sponge is like the paper towels. Since this is erectile tissue, its size varies depending on the level of arousal. When the sponge hasn't been stimulated, it's like you're at the end of the roll. When the sponge gets the attention it so richly deserves, it engorges and becomes like a brand-new jumbo roll.

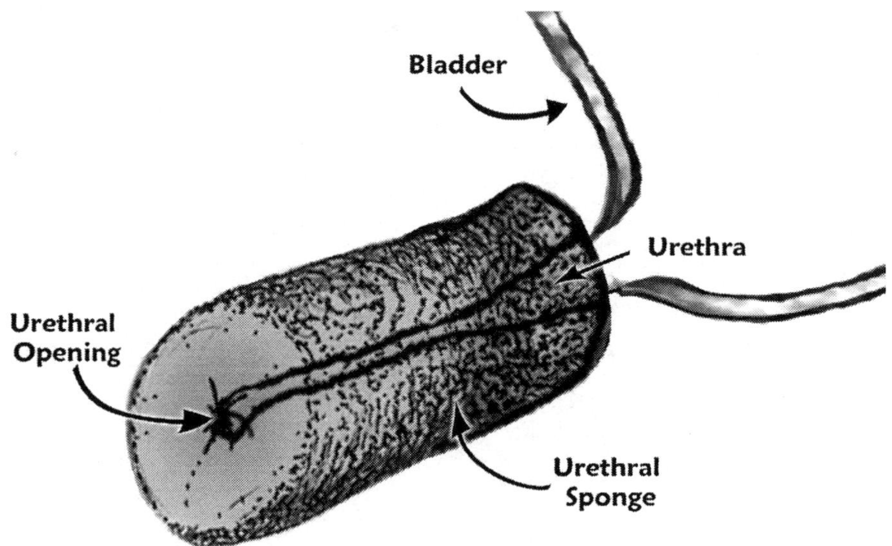

The Urethral Sponge

Whether you're a visitor or the owner, you'll find that it's much easier to appreciate the urethral sponge's size, shape, contour and erotic potential after it's engorged. When un-engorged, the urethral sponge is difficult to see or feel. In this state, stimulation will often feel irritating and can make the owner feel like she needs to pee. However, playing with the sponge after the woman is at high-level arousal will often be appreciated. (Very appreciated!)

If playing with it doesn't feel fabulous, retreat. Get to deeper, more thorough arousal first, then go back to exploring the pleasure potential of this part of the erectile matrix. In general, the urethral sponge responds to firm, rhythmic stimulation.

In addition to being part of the erectile network, the urethral sponge serves another function. It houses the paraurethral glands—the source of

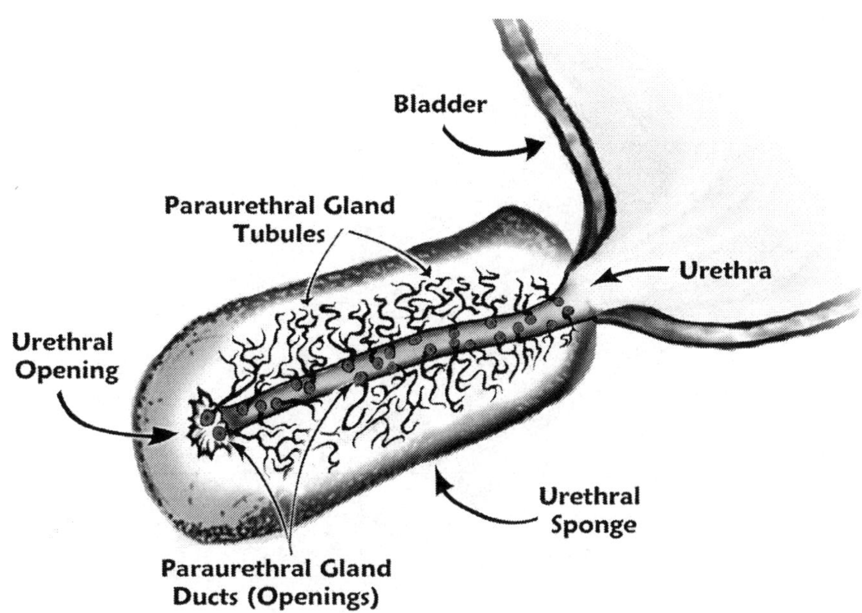

The Paraurethral Glands

female ejaculate. Although there isn't scientific consensus on this point, I'm convinced this fluid is part of the immune system and that it helps protect women from urinary tract infections.

While not all women 'she-jaculate' profusely, I believe all women produce at least a small amount of fluid during arousal. Some women are 'natural ejaculators'—they always gush at some point in arousal or with orgasm. For other women, obvious and abundant ejaculation is a learned experience—they've discovered how to squirt and to amplify their gushability. As discussed at length in Chapter 12, every woman has the capacity to make significant amounts of ejaculate and can learn to release it. It's an amazing sensation: Copious gushing, especially in concert with orgasm, feels intensely sacred and ecstatic.

We're still not done. There's one more wad of female genital erectile tissue, the perineal sponge (or perineal body). It lies under the floor of the vagina, in the wall between the vaginal and anal canals. You'll find it about an inch, more or less, inside the anal sphincter or vagina—you can access it from either opening. Like the urethral sponge, this erectile tissue responds best when its owner is already at high-level arousal. For most women, the perineal sponge responds to firm strokes and squeezes and deep pressure.

When all the parts of the female erectile network are aroused, they form a circuit of delightfully swollen erectile tissue—a 'she-rection.' For a woman to achieve her prodigious pleasure potential, get every bit of this snug, expandable erectile cuff totally stimulated.

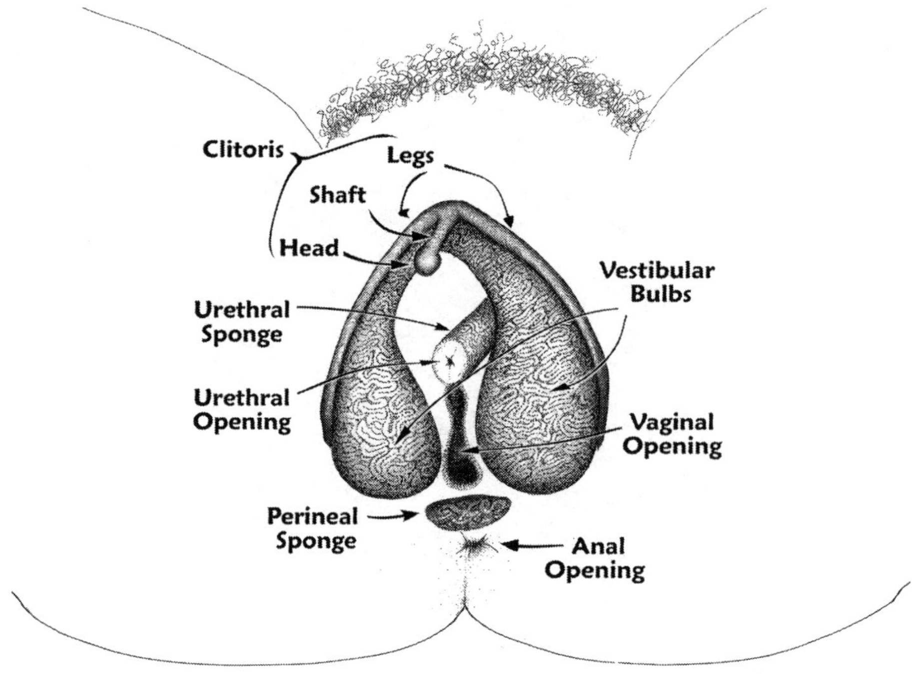

The Female Erectile Network

Unlike penises, which are more of an all-or-nothing apparatus, some parts of the female erectile network can be engorged while others remain flaccid. If you don't play with each of the structures, they may not swell. Only when you attend to all the pieces of the engorgeable equipment do you get the full circuit of connected structures along with the spectacular effects of the connections—a deep, thorough arousal trance and easier access to the woman's full orgasmic potential.

The simple and sad truth is that because so few people know about most of the parts of the female erectile network, many sexual encounters fall far short

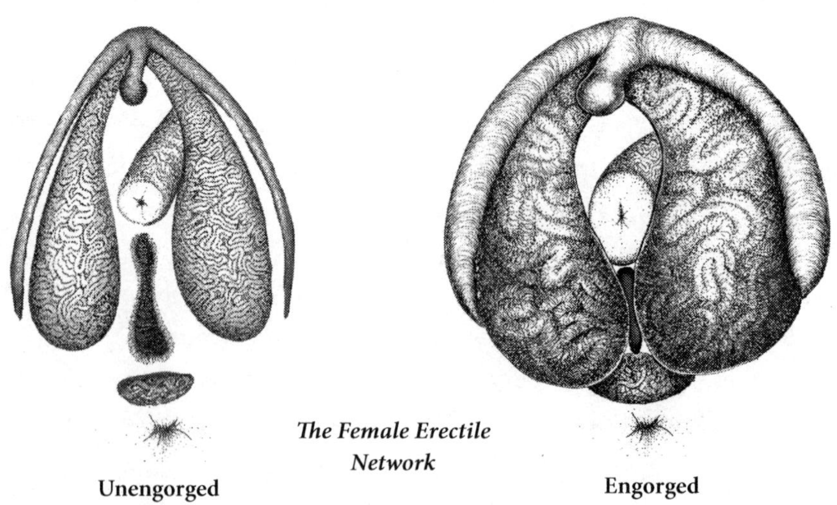

The Female Erectile Network

of what they might be. Clitoral stimulation is a fine and usually necessary part of female arousal and orgasm—it's just not the only thing you can turn on. Puffing up the entire female erectile network makes it much easier to have vaginal, multiple and extended orgasms.

Women, do yourselves a big favor and get to know your female erectile network better. Spend some quality time having solo dates to explore your equipment. Play with yourself, ideally with a mirror at hand, and note how things feel and look before you're aroused and then at medium and high arousal. It's a fun and fabulous journey of discovery.

Lovers of women, there's also a big payoff for you in learning your way around the female erectile network. Driving a Chevy is fun. So is driving a Mustang. But wouldn't you rather be driving a Lamborghini?

Penises, Prostates and Perineums, Oh My!

While men's sexual anatomy doesn't harbor a hidden matrix of erectile tissue, some aspects of the male equipment can benefit from a closer look (and feel).

Like vulvas—and faces, and flowers— penises span a wide range in size, shape and color. The realm of normal is vast—and they're all created equal. Despite what our culture tells us, bigger is not better. Most people who like to play with penises enjoy a variety of sizes. Some people do have clear preferences, often for penises that fit their particular orifices best. Some partners love modestly-sized penises, some prefer really big ones and most enjoy the wide range of mediums out there.

Guys, having a bigger member doesn't make you a better lover or more of a man. Some women actually find big penises a problem because they're uncomfortable. Having a magnum can also shrink the palette of possible activities—a supersized man may be unwelcome at the anus, for instance. I'm not saying it's a bad thing to be big, but it doesn't make you a stud either, not unless you're with a size queen. All in all, it's not what you have but what you do with it and—more importantly—with the rest of you that counts.

Whatever its size, a penis has three sections—the top end called the *head* or *glans*, the mid-section called the *shaft* (*body* or *corpus*), and the base (the *root* or *bulb*). The *glans* is the helmet-shaped head. The rim at the base of the glans is the sensitive *corona*. If you have a foreskin, when you draw it back you'll see the Y-shaped elastic tissue bridge of the *frenulum* (just like the one under our tongues). The frenulum is highly sensitive and is mostly removed by circumcision. For circumcised men, what's left of it is often a lovely spot for stimulation. The head and the shaft of the penis have no shortage of ways they like being pleasured, so I'll not detail them here. (The next chapter, by Carlyle Jansen on oral sex, offers lovely options.)

The root is the part of the penis that's attached to the body—while the shaft is the part that hangs loose. Here's a little-known fact: One-third to one-half the penis is anchored—only a part of the penis dangles free. That's right, guys, your magic wand is up to 100% bigger than you thought it was! (Not that size matters.) Still, the connected part of the penis is an oft-ignored and sizable mass of highly pleasurable erectile tissue. Penis-pleasurers, I encourage you to give the root the attention it deserves. You can access it through the skin of the scrotum and from the area that's just below and behind the testicles.

Our next landmark in penis geography, the foreskin, is a tricky one. For many men, especially in the US, it's a missing piece of the penis puzzle. Due to the common and unfortunate practice of male circumcision, many men are lacking this functionally important and highly pleasurable part of their equipment.*

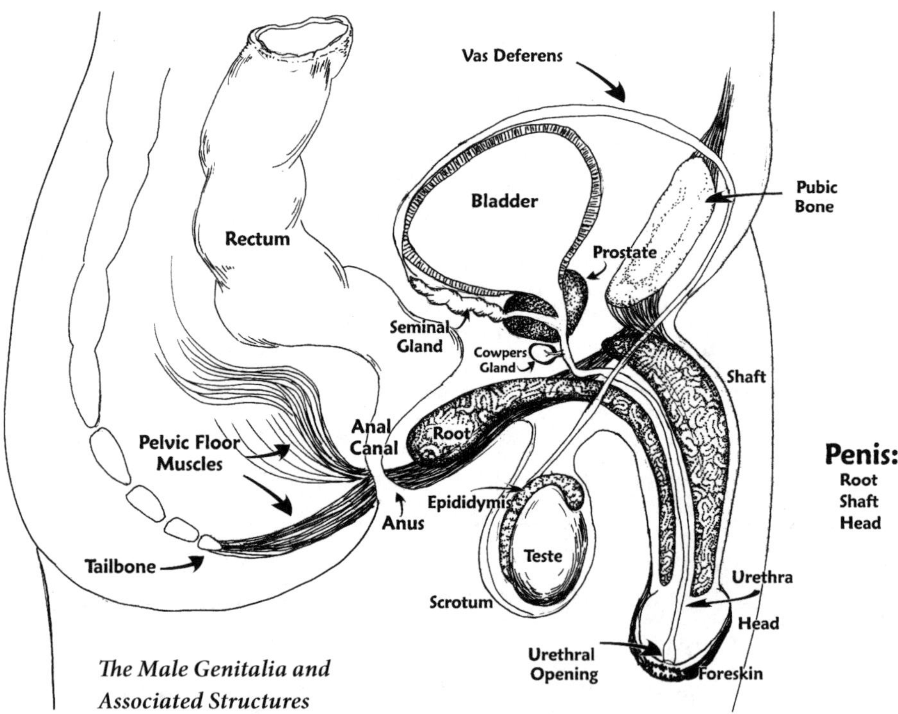

The Male Genitalia and Associated Structures

The foreskin is the most sensitive part of the male sexual apparatus. Rather than being a separate structure, it's an integral part of the penis. A foreskin is a double-layered continuation of the sliding skin system that extends over the whole penis. When flaccid, the foreskin covers the head. During erection,

* The foreskin has over a dozen different functions relating to pleasure and health. My hope is that if we have a better understanding of what a foreskin is and what it's for, we will stop doing circumcisions and offer future generations of boys an intact body.

it everts—the inner layer rolls outward, moving to the exterior. Inside the foreskin is a stretchy elastic inner ring that contains super-sensitive nerve endings. They respond very happily to stretching and stroking sensations as the sleeve rolls back and forth over the head and are one of the primary orgasmic triggers in uncircumcised men.

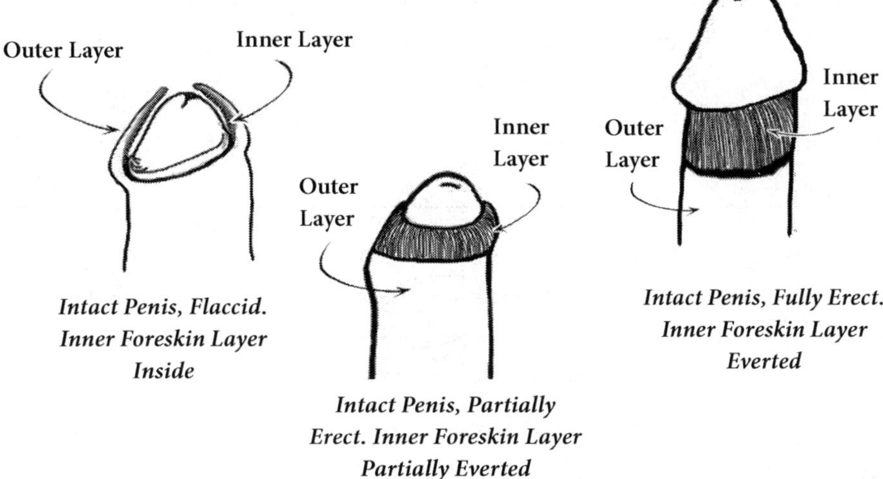

Intact Penis, Flaccid. Inner Foreskin Layer Inside

Intact Penis, Partially Erect. Inner Foreskin Layer Partially Everted

Intact Penis, Fully Erect. Inner Foreskin Layer Everted

While not every man in our culture has a foreskin, almost every man does have another source of potential erotic delight. Moving inside the male body, we find the walnut-sized *prostate gland* surrounding the base of the urethra. The prostate has two lobes with a cleft running between them. The urethra passes through the prostate, much like the female urethra passes through the urethral sponge.* Like its female counterpart the urethral sponge, the prostate is composed of both erectile and glandular tissue. It produces prostate fluid, which is a component of semen.

The prostate is very sensitive and can deliver enormous pleasure. However, because of its internal location, it doesn't get the respect or attention it deserves. By far the best way to play with it involves anal access, so an unfortunately large number of men consider it off limits, being afflicted with the notion that being on the receiving end of anal play may mean they're gay. If you're one of these naysayers, I encourage you to change your story. Enjoying anal play says nothing whatsoever about your sexual preferences. (Except for this—you like anal play!) Prostate stimulation can deliver new sensations, expanded arousal and amazing orgasms, it can help you learn to have non-ejaculatory orgasms—and it's really healthy for you!

*** Embryologically, the prostate and urethral sponge arise from the same tissue. Thus the urethral sponge can accurately be referred to as the female prostate, and conversely, the prostate could be called the male urethral sponge.**

If you aren't a prostate player yet, I invite you to get bold and go for it. As with any new activity, I encourage you to try it out in your solo play with the aid of specially-designed toys. On the other hand, so to speak, you may know someone who'll provide a friendly finger. (For prostate pleasuring ideas, see Chapter 3.)

Returning to the outside of the body, we come to the perineum, the stretch of skin between the southerly edges of the genitals and the opening of the ass. Although both men and women have a perineum, I'm discussing it here because it's where a number of male pleasure points are located. As mentioned earlier, you can access the attached base of the penis from the perineum. With very firm pressure, you can stimulate the prostate, albeit somewhat indirectly. Also, the spot just behind the base of the penis is renowned in Taoist sexuality teachings as the *million dollar point.* When you press on it, it taps into a powerful masculine sexual energy current. You can play with the deep pulsation that arises there to great effect.

The secrets of male genital anatomy aren't as dramatic as the female ones, but it's still useful to know about the uncelebrated parts and how to make them happy. Familiarity will help you please your male sex partners better—and if you happen to own the equipment, understanding your anatomy more deeply is a first step on the road to advanced skills like full-body and non-ejaculatory orgasms. (Male non-ejaculatory orgasm is discussed in Chapter 11.)

Energy Polarity

Which comes first, energy or anatomy? In this chapter, I discussed anatomy first, but not because it's more important. If anything, the opposite is true. Passion and ecstasy don't only emerge from the physical contact of bodies. It's the *energetic* connection that really sets off the fireworks—the magnetic attraction of powerful dynamic currents.

Erotic energy is a manifestation of the life force. How we channel it through our bodies is ultimately what makes sex so amazing and powerful.

So which comes first? Energy. The body comes along for the ride.

In Chapter 15, we'll explore playing with your erotic energy. Here, we're focusing on *polarity*—the manifestation of two opposite or contrasting principles or tendencies.

Our world and all life are composed of a dynamic interplay of polarities. These energies aren't in opposition—they're complementary and require each other. To see, we need both light and dark. Without illumination, we'd be stumbling around in the dark. Without shadows to give us contours and edges, we'd have only blinding light. Neither is better or worse than the other.

They don't clash, they co-exist. Together these polarities create the dynamic homeostasis that is life. You consume and excrete, inhale and exhale, wake and sleep. There's day and night, matter and energy, masculine and feminine and all the other dualities. At the micro level, atomic particles have positive and negative forces that attract and repel, that bond and release. At the macro level, our planet is polarized by its north and south poles. Somewhere in between, you were created by a sperm and an egg.

These polarities are universal forces that pull and push in the dynamic, eternal dance of life, including the forces that create attraction, desire and the urge to mate and merge.

Core and Complement

Broadly stated, there are two kinds of energy in the world (and us). In the Taoist tradition the hot, steady fire of the sun is the initiatory, active, focused energy of *yang*. The cool, fluid, watery energy of the moon is the fluctuating, receptive, creative energy of *yin*. As we've seen, the polarities aren't in opposition—they're two ends of a spectrum.

Although we all have both yin and yang within us, when it comes to sexuality, most people have a dominant polarity. This stronger energetic tendency forms their core energy. Your core energy is your default position—it's where you tend to start from and where you go more often. It's your more natural preference. It usually manifests in our sexual expression (what we like to do and have done to us) and attracts us to those with the opposite core polarity.

If one polarity is your stronger core way of being, than the opposite pole is your secondary, complementary energy. Your complementary energy balances and leavens your dominant aspect. Although it is your peripheral, less powerful energy, it's no less important than your core. To be healthy and internally balanced, your primary core energy needs to be counter-balanced by your secondary aspect.

Speaking in 'genderalities,' we commonly associate yang energy with 'masculine' qualities. Yang is the core energy and primary quality of most (but not all) men. It's often (but not always) the secondary, complementary energy of women.* Yin is associated with qualities that we commonly think of as feminine. Yin is the core energy of most (but not all) women. It's usually

*** Talking in generalities about male and female sexuality is tricky territory. For one thing, for any generalizations there are always exceptions. For another, generalizations about gender and sexuality can be limiting, sexist and offensive. Please remember that we're talking about energy here, not anatomy. Masculine and feminine energy are cosmic and eternal forces and not at all political. Sexual politics matter—a lot. But they're not relevant here.**

(but not always) the complementary energy for folks with male bodies. For a minority of people, these energetic patterns and the associated male or female plumbing are reversed, while a small number of people have equal amounts of yin and yang. All these ways of being energetically wired are normal. There's no right or wrong, no better or worse. The only thing that matters here is understanding your energetic tendencies and those of your partner(s) so you can play nicely and skillfully together.

The Dance of Yin and Yang

Yin energy is slow, cool and watery. Like a river, it flows and fluctuates.

It's also associated with darkness, the night and the moon. These qualities have been associated with women since time immemorial because of the very real link between women's fertility cycles and the changing moon. Although it's less so now due to the advent of electric lights and other factors, in primal cultures women's menstrual cycles were closely linked to the moon phase. Like the moon, feminine energy is always waxing and waning. It fluctuates, shifting from expansion to contraction, growing and diminishing in a cyclic pattern. Women are changeable because they do in fact go through numerous transformations. The fluctuations of menarche, the menstrual cycle, pregnancy, birth, postpartum, breast-feeding and menopause all come with the territory, so to speak, of women's sexuality.

Yin energy also has the quality of opening and closing. When open, yin receives and radiates invitation. When closed, she can contract, clam up and deny permission to enter.

At the root of yin energy is the longing to open all the way and to surrender utterly. This cannot be forced. The owners of yin body parts like the vulva and the ass can allow them to open (and their visitors can encourage it), but no one can make them open.

Yin energy also has a deep and special magic to it—the power of transformation. As the feminine principle, yin makes magic manifest with her miraculous power of creation, gestation and birth. Yin receives (inspiration, sperm, energy) and cooks it up in her cauldron of transformation. She then showers forth abundance in the form of love, *amrita* (the sacred name for female ejaculate), a child, and every other ecstatic form of creation.

All acts of creativity use yin magic. Regardless of your plumbing, if you're creating and then birthing your creation, you're using your yin power.

Yang energy is commonly associated with qualities we think of as masculine. Steady and stalwart, it's the energy of fire and light. Yang energy is fast, fiery and focused. It's the power of the sun and the consistent circadian daily rhythm.

Yang is initiatory. It's about direction, about moving in and out, or towards and away. Yang penetrates, inserts, puts forth. It loves to be doing. It seeks to fix, to accomplish, to work, and ultimately to serve. It desires to penetrate the world with action, to offer its gifts and assert (and insert) its influence.

Great partner sex is a playful improvisation of yang giving and yin receiving.

Yang energy is the container, the form that gives shape to the flow, like the banks of the stream that keep the water from flooding. It provides the structure within which spontaneity can arise. In dancing the tango, it's the lead dancer (traditionally but not necessarily male) who provides the container and the direction within which his partner flows.

Yang is the energy that drives the archetypes of the Guardian who protects and the Warrior who defends the vulnerable and defenseless.

The sexual polarity of yin and yang creates the exhilarating dance of attraction and mating that fuels our desire to connect and to merge, to enter or be filled, to play in the fields of erotic delight.

We each have both aspects within us. Masculine and feminine, yin and yang, estrogen and testosterone, fire and water, sun and moon, we each contain them all. And, while we may spend more time inhabiting our core polarity, everyone shifts back and forth and embodies both polarities at different times. In fact, great partner sex is a playful improvisation of yang giving and yin receiving.

Yin and Yang in the Bedroom

Both yin and yang energies have characteristic qualities and patterns that help us understand how they like to play and be played with.

Yin energy goes from out to in. It begins outside the person in the context and the quality of the connection between people. The energy then moves to the edges, slowly shifting to the center. If you want to relate to a yin being, start with creating connection. Be patient as her energy takes time to move inward and coalesce in her sex centers.

Yin energy starts cool and is slow to heat up. She takes awhile to come to a boil, but once the water's roiling, she can stay hot for a long time. If yin energy is ignored and shut down, its cool quality can get cold and even freeze. That's why it's important for core yin folks to fire up their erotic energy on a more or less consistent basis.

That's right—if you're a core yin person, the best way to keep your sexual juice flowing is to use it regularly. And take your time doing so. If you're suffering from low libido or very slow arousal, you can ramp up your desire by getting stimulated and aroused on a fairly consistent basis—it'll turn on your desire to desire. The more often you boil your water, the easier it will be to fire it up again. The less often you heat your energy, the likelier it is to get frozen.

What yin longs for most is to release her boundaries, to open wide and receive fully. She yearns to give up control. But she needs to feel safe in order to do so. When yin dissolves in surrender and ecstasy, it's beautiful to behold.

If you have a yin partner, the best way to turn her on is by not heading directly toward your goal. The better approach is like piloting a sailboat—you have to take the boat, the sails, the water currents and the wind into account. You rarely go straight to the destination. Instead you tack back and forth as you work with the water and wind, finessing your way across the bay. While you're still 'yangly' focused on the ultimate destination, you understand that the fastest way to get there is by honoring the yin nature of your partner and following the cues of her desire. The path you take today won't be the same as the one you'll use tomorrow when the currents and the weather are different. Each journey is attuned to the unique conditions of the moment. (And, of course, the uniqueness of the boat.)

For core yang folks, arousal starts with the genital ignition switch. While other sex centers in the brain are also activated during initial yang arousal (specifically, the "yum, that looks good!" brain region), the predominant energetic focal point is usually the genitals (typically a penis). This explains the common pattern in men (or any primarily yang person) to become quickly and easily aroused. Yang energy is like a fire in dry tinder. It's quick to ignite and if not husbanded carefully, quick to consume its fuel and burn out. Core yang folk need to learn to keep their fire burning long enough to boil their yin-partner's water. They'll also increase their own pleasure by learning to steward and spread their yang energy.

In a pattern that's opposite to yin, yang begins at the center and travels out. For yang people, their arousal typically starts genitally and moves outward from there, either with a quick short genital ejaculation that erupts out from the penis or, if they've learned how to moderate and channel the energy, in a slower, more whole-body orgasmic experience.

Yang loves to head straight for the goal, much like steering a motorboat directly toward its destination. You're focused on your objective and zoom right for it, swift as an arrow aiming for its target. If you partner with core yang people, they'll usually appreciate it when you dive right in to their genitals. And stay there for a good long time!

As we've seen, yang energy provides the focus, discipline and direction that enables yin creativity to take shape and manifest. It's the channel for the current. Core yang (or anyone in a yang mood) longs to serve yin, to provide the cauldron for her ecstatic magic. Yang loves to be the one that's responsible for—and gets to watch—their yin partners dissolve in rapture. Yum!

Yang At Its Best—Appropriate, Attuned and Attentive Giving

What does it look like when you have a healthy inner equilibrium with your primary core power balanced by your secondary complementary force? That depends on if your core is yin or yang.

Yang energy is about containing, initiating, and penetrating, about actively inserting, about pushing something out into the world. When yang's penetrating force is complemented by healthy and well-developed yin energy, it gives rise to *appropriate, attuned and attentive giving.* It's about giving your partner exactly what they want, exactly how and when they want it, about penetrating your partner with love, about using your direction and focus to put your gift out to those that want and need it. Ultimately, it's about being in service, contributing what is most desired and needed—to yourself, your partner and the world. You offer your service, provide focus and direction and do what needs to be done by penetrating the planet (or your partner) with love and attention.

Imagine for a moment that you want to befriend a beautiful kitty (an excellent exemplar of yin energy). You are the yang pursuer. Are you all yang, all the time without the leavening force of your own complementary energy? Do you run up and grab her, force her onto her back and rub her tummy? For both your sake and the cat's, I hope not. You're much likelier to succeed if you use your complementary yin energy to pay attention to her signals. Did you miss the warning signs of her ears back and her swishing annoyed tail? If you tried to grab her anyway, you were not being appropriate and attuned. You'd probably end up bleeding and she'd be out of there. You'd have a hard time getting a second chance at that pussy! Fail!

Of course, you know better. You use your yang mellowed by yin, your appropriate attuned attention. You start by creating connection. You get her interest and make eye contact. Since yin pussycats can only relax and open when they feel secure, she checks you out to see if you're safe. You approach her slowly, attending to her responses. You notice if she's opening in interest or closing and withdrawing. If you go at the right pace—her pace—at some point you'll get to pet her. You wisely start with the less vulnerable parts of her body. You watch her signals. You give her pleasure, but not too much. Don't overwhelm her or move too fast to her tender parts. If you're very clever, you'll arouse her desire. Pet and rub her just a little bit less then she wants—

then she'll want more. Take your time, prove you're safe and can be trusted to give pleasure. If you pet her the way she loves to be petted, sooner or later you'll have the purring puddle of pussy you've been hoping for.

Yin At Its Best—Active, Conscious Reception

While unbalanced yin is exemplified by the doormat, when yin is balanced by yang it's not at all passive. You can be a yin flower without being a wall flower. When core yin is balanced, contained and fortified by healthy well-developed secondary yang, you have *active, conscious reception*. You choose who and what you open for.

Yin infused with yang enables you to make conscious choices about who is allowed entry into your most sacred parts—about who deserves the privilege of being your playmate. In order to allow yourself to open and surrender to their penetration, you need to trust your inner guardian to make wise choices. You need to feel safe. With a partner, in order to get to the place of dissolving in ecstatic surrender, you need to hand over control of your nervous system. It's like letting someone else drive your car. You can relax when you trust that they know how to drive safely and can get you where you want to go. In fact, if they're a truly fabulous driver, you can totally surrender and they can take you places that you may have never dreamed it was possible to get to. Your own guardian needs to be satisfied that you've chosen well and have a trustworthy partner who is in attuned and attentive service to your pleasure. Then you can relax and let them drive.

When you consciously choose to open and receive, you can do so actively, sucking in delightedly like a snake ingesting delicious prey. You can receive enthusiastically and voraciously. Yang lovers, I ask you: Is there anything hotter than hungry receptivity? Yin partners, is there anything hotter than a lover who you trust to take you all the way out?

Ultimately all of us can access every aspect of both these polarities. We can all be all of these things, for ourselves and our playmates.

To be a really skilled lover, bring both your primary and secondary aspects into play. You won't want to be too yang-aggressive (that's the rapist) or too yin-passive (that's the doormat, the victim). Be an attuned and attentive giver, and receive with an active appetite. And while you will probably spend the majority of your time in your dominant polarity, don't forget to dance into your secondary polarity, too.

If you can be present and play in this way while also applying what you've learned about genital anatomy, you're well on your way to being a sex master.

SEXY SUMMARY

THE BETTER YOU UNDERSTAND genital anatomy—and apply your knowledge—the farther into ecstasy you'll be able to go and take your partner.

WOMEN HAVE A SET OF CONNECTED STRUCTURES composed of erectile tissue—the female erectile network. For full female arousal, get the whole network activated.

NEGLECTED OR ABSENT ASPECTS of the male apparatus include the foreskin, prostate and the root of the penis.

IN THE DANCE OF SEX, which also just happens to be the dance of life, there are two main forces—feminine (or yin) energy and masculine (or yang) energy. Erotic warm-up unfolds very differently within these systems. Yin warms up slowly and is variable, so take your time and be present to what's happening in the moment. Yang warms up quickly and is pretty predictable. What worked yesterday will probably work again today. Also, yin energy moves from the outside in. You'll want to work up to it—more precisely, you'll want to work them up to it—before playing with the genitals. Yang is different—have at 'em!

PLAY WITH YOUR PARTNERS in ways that honor their natural polarity.

USE YOUR DOMINANT and secondary polarities in your erotic improvs.

CARLYLE JANSEN *is a sex coach, sex educator, writer and video blogger. She is the founder of Good For Her, Toronto's premiere sexuality shop and workshop center, and producer of the annual Feminist Porn Awards. Since 1995, Carlyle has been teaching workshops about sexual pleasure and sexuality and coaching individuals and couples to help them enhance their sexual lives. She is an invited speaker for medical, health and sexuality professionals at events such as the Intensive Sex Therapy Training program.*

Carlyle's areas of focus include sexual technique and pleasure, youth education, sex and parenting, and sexual challenges. She works with individuals and couples in person and over Skype and Facetime to help them find more pleasure, desire and intimacy in their sexual lives.

You can find her and her work at CarlyleJansen.com. You can also follow her on Facebook and twitter as Carlyle Jansen.

Her free video blogs are on Youtube at goodforherdotcom.

CHAPTER TWO

Sensational Oral Sex

by Carlyle Jansen

ART BY AMY NOSEWORTHY

ORAL SEX IS ONE OF THOSE DELICACIES THAT TRULY IS A GIFT since we can't give it to ourselves, though many have tried. Numerous people do it as a matter of course while others reserve it for special occasions or leave it off the menu entirely. Some consider it not 'real' sex or not a big deal to perform. Most people, though, consider it a very intimate activity. Wherever you happen to be on the turn-on/turn-off continuum, you probably have strong feelings about oral sex—it's rarely something people feel neutral about. Maybe you love to give, but resist getting. Maybe it's the reverse—or maybe you love, dislike or even detest both.

Despite the considerable progress that's occurred in recent decades, oral sex continues to be culturally fraught. Many have received mixed messages about oral pleasure from society, culture, friends, family and partners, often leaving them with physical or emotional hurdles to overcome. Whatever your beliefs or blocks, oral sex can be a wonderful way to connect and to give and receive amazing pleasure. First, though, you might need to address any feelings of shame, contempt or being disrespected that it brings up for you.

Cultural Norms and Personal Inhibitions

Cultural norms about oral sex are wildly varied, both pro and con. Some people view going down as unremarkable, healthy or as we've seen, barely sex at all. Others are repelled by the mere thought of oral sex because it seems unnatural or unclean. And then there's the famous double standard, with heterosexual oral sex on one gender (usually the man) viewed as okay while going down on a woman is seen as emasculating and uncool. ("Real men don't do that.")

Another obstacle is the belief that only promiscuous, 'un-ladylike' women would stoop—literally— to putting their mouths on someone else's genitals. While nothing obligates anyone to perform oral sex, it's a shame if the reluctance stems from sex-negative biases or norms.

Yet another misplaced assumption is that oral sex is foreplay, something to be done before intercourse. While there's nothing wrong with this sequence, it's limiting to treat oral sex as only the hors d'oeuvre. Many women enjoy oral sex more than penetration and reach orgasm more easily that way. There's nothing wrong with having oral sex be your final destination.

From one perspective, it's irrational not to enjoy receiving oral pleasure. Why not lie back and be showered with whatever indulgences a partner wishes to lavish on you? When it comes to sex (and much else), we're not entirely rational, though. When receiving their partner's undivided oral attention, some people feel self-conscious, embarrassed or afraid they'll seem selfish. Sometimes our guilt gets the better of us and we feel called upon to pleasure our partner simultaneously.

If you're one of the many people who has bought into society's many incorrect and sex-negative messages that our genitals—especially our vulvas—are dirty, smelly, ugly and taste terrible, you might feel even more self-conscious, as if you are putting a partner through the awful torture of pleasuring you orally. How many of us have at some point decided to put our partner out of their 'misery' (although they may be having a fabulous time) by giving them 'the tap' and moving onto something more mutual, like intercourse? This happens all the time, even though this choice often leads to less pleasure. Whatever messages you may have imbibed, the reality is that you are doing yourself and your partner a service by settling back and enjoying being pleasured orally. Lots of people love to dine south of the border. As the receiver, all you need to do is take them at their word and enjoy being feasted upon.

Just as some of us are uneasy about receiving oral sex, others are reluctant to give it. We may have cleanliness concerns or not like the taste. It may seem strange and unnatural. We may have bought into the line about "Good girls (or real men) don't do that." All these negative attitudes can be overcome—if you choose to. Doing this requires you to get more comfortable with bodies in general and to dismantle any negative stories you might have about giving and getting head. There's nothing unnatural or unclean about oral sex, and genitals are a totally appropriate and sexy object of oral desire. If you're having trouble embracing these beliefs, a sex-positive friend or therapist can help.

That said, it's also the case that you shouldn't feel under any duty to give or get oral sex. Choosing not to go there is always a valid option and needs to be respected.

A Matter of Taste

Do you have issues with the taste or texture of body fluids? We can probably all agree that sexual juices aren't chocolate. Whatever your equipment, your taste down there is earthy, salty and intense. For many, genital juices are an acquired taste, like wine. But lots of people love to quaff the grape, and lots of people love to give head, too.

If you don't like your partner's taste today, don't despair—they may have another flavor tomorrow. People taste different at different times. Factors include their overall diet, what they ate in the last few hours, when they last showered, and (if she's a pre-menopausal woman) where she is in her menstrual cycle.

If you want to get comfortable with how genital fluids taste, there's one person you can always get a sample from—yourself! Seriously: If you want to get comfortable with 'that' taste, get some moisture from your vulva or put a dab of your own ejaculate on your tongue and find out how it tastes. (Don't worry, it won't change your sexual orientation!) It may not ever become your favorite flavor of all time, but the chances are excellent that, with continued sampling and the intention to enjoy it, it'll come to taste tolerable or even better. In fact, you may eventually decide that even if it's not the best flavor in the world, it certainly is the sexiest!

It's easy for considerate receivers to freshen themselves up for an oral sex date. Showering with water is all you need. Add a little ph-balanced soap if you wish, but as long as you get water into all your folds and crevices, you'll be clean as a whistle. Givers, if you prefer squeaky-clean, I encourage you to speak up. Do so courteously and considerately—but speak up. If you are concerned about how your partner might react, suggest a sexy shower or bath for the two of you together. By spending extra time seductively cleaning your partner's genitals, you can transform an unpleasant experience into a delightful one.

Another consideration is diet. If you want your juices to be sweeter, eat pineapple, strawberry, apple, pear, kiwi, melon or celery. Things to avoid include alcohol, vitamins, asparagus, beets, coffee, cigarettes and garlic. (Sorry!)

Sometimes a person worries that they don't taste 'normal' even though they do (whatever 'normal' means!). If this is the case, I encourage the giver to reassure them. Tell them they taste great and how much fun you're having. If you want, go the extra mile and tell them there's absolutely no rush and that you'd be quite happy to linger down there for hours. While they may not completely believe you, it'll make it easier for them to surrender to the wonders of your mouth and tongue. People don't want you to be bored or uncomfortable, they don't want to feel selfish and they don't want to feel distasteful (literally). Reassuring them helps shoo away these negative thoughts and has the extra benefit of reinforcing your positive feelings as well.

Porn Delusions

You might think pornography would help people get over oral sex concerns, but the opposite is more often true. Porn doesn't make it easier to get down with going down because what's shown isn't realistic. If we were to take what we see in pornography as gospel, we'd assume that penises are easy to deep-throat and that it all it takes to get a woman to come is to lick like a lizard on the head of her clit for a few seconds.

It's not so fast and it's not so easy. Penises, including smaller-sized ones, are quite large objects to put into our mouths. Gagging is a reflex: It can happen when you put anything in the back of your mouth, and it doesn't have to be a penis—it could be a toothbrush. Unless you're ready to do some special training, gagging is pretty much guaranteed if you try to take your partner's penis into your throat.

While it's a great skill to learn, it's also important to remember that you don't have to do deep throat to give fantastic fellatio. Ask any guy and they'll tell you that pretty much any mouth- and tongue-related action on their penis feels good. With a little practice and imagination, it's easy to move the dial from good to great. Deep throat is a challenging, super-deluxe—and not mandatory—treat. Don't feel obligated to do it.

As for cunnilingus, most vulva owners appreciate being pleasured with much more than just the tip of the tongue. It is sometimes called "giving face" (not giving head) because once the pussy is warmed up, the giver's entire face can be used to provide pleasure.

What looks good on camera (where actors often fake their pleasure) is very different from what people tend to like most in real life. Don't be intimidated by porn performers and don't compete with them, either. Let your own experience and your partner's pleasure guide you.

What's Good for the Goose *and* Good for the Gander

Let's look at some general principles that apply regardless of what type of plumbing you're pleasuring.

A Note About Sexually Transmitted Infections (STIs)

While oral sex is generally considered low risk for HIV/AIDS, it is medium- to high-risk for syphilis, gonorrhea, herpes and HPV (human papilloma virus). Ways to practice safer oral sex include:

- Don't brush or floss immediately prior to giving oral sex. These otherwise hygienic activities create small open wounds inside the mouth that make it easier for unwanted bacteria and viruses to enter the bloodstream.
- Use a dental dam for cunnilingus, especially if the woman on the receiving end is menstruating, which increases the risk of HIV transmission. (It's healthy, normal and fun to go down on a menstruating vulva—just be more careful about STIs.)
- Use a condom for fellatio. This is the Official Recommendation and it's there for good reason. But it's also true that if you're going to put a somewhat unknown penis somewhere in your body without a condom, the mouth is safer than your anus or vagina. If there's no way you'll suck a cock while it's covered, the next best level of precaution is to not deep-throat. The back of the throat is more susceptible to infection than the mouth.

While using a dental dam or condom can take some of the fun away, there are ways to maximize the pleasure for both parties, as discussed in Eve Minax's chapter on eroticizing safer sex.

First: Communicate. Ask your partner what they like—and do this when you're not having sex. Unless you're amazingly flexible, it's really difficult to demonstrate on yourself what you like, so during your pre-sex conversations feel free to use a prop like a cucumber, dildo, peach or vulva toy, especially if your partner has different plumbing.

It's especially important to communicate with women about what they like because their preferences differ considerably—and, in addition, what works for a woman often varies depending on her mood, menstrual cycle and other factors. Feel free to pause from time to time to poke your head up like a prairie dog and ask, "Do you like this? How is the pressure?" It never hurts to check in.

It's also a good idea to check in with the woman before going down on her because it can be hard to hear her answers when your ears are smooshed against her thighs.

If your bedmate asks for more or less pressure, do as they ask and check in to see if your softer is soft enough or your harder is hard enough. Most people won't make the same request twice, so it's important to follow their communication lead the first time.

In the heat of the bedroom, it's a good idea to ask simple questions so your partner doesn't have to do much processing to answer—having to go into thinking mode distracts the receiver from their pleasure. Questions that can be answered with one word are better than ones that require the incredibly arduous task of stringing words into sentences. "Is this about right?" "Do you want it harder? Do you want it softer?" Because these questions require only a yes-no answer, they're great for the tripped-out person whose blood is mostly in their genitals.

If your partner isn't communicative about their preferences—and this does happen—try to read their body language. Let their breathing, body movements and sounds guide you in deciphering whether or not what you're doing is pleasing them.

Second: If you're settling in for a long meal, get comfortable—both of you. It's hard to receive fully or give skilfully if you're hurting. If she's on her back, put her in a semi-fetal position with her knees up to her chest. This will take the stress off your neck and makes it easier for you to access all her pelvic erogenous zones. If he is standing, don't numb your legs by kneeling. Sit on something low like a footstool or bottom stair so you can be relaxed and enjoy the process.

Third and fourth: Two equal opportunity techniques that delight both penises and vulvas are humming and blowing. Humming creates a vibration that adds pleasure to the receiver. If you've got a soundtrack playing, you can hum along to the music, or you can make a sound like "mmm." You'll get a double benefit from this: Your partner will feel the exciting vibrations and also be reassured and aroused by your sounds of pleasure as the giver.

Blowing air is equally easy (and gentle). First, make the penis or vulva wet, either by licking it or adding lube—this heightens the sensation. Try taking a long lick up the side of the penis or from bottom to top of the labia, followed by a gentle exhalation as if you were slowly blowing out a candle. This produces a pleasurably cool sensation. Want to warm it up? Open your mouth wider and blow from the back of your throat, the way you would to warm up your hands in winter.

Finally, enjoy! Sex is supposed to be fun for everyone, and that means the giver as well as the receiver. If you're not into it, this lack of enthusiasm will transmit to your partner and they'll have less fun, too. So get creative, try some of the techniques listed in this chapter, make sure it's working for your partner, and revel in what you're doing!

The Ups and Downs of Sixty-Nine

Oral sex is great both ways, but not always simultaneously. Sixty-nine is like communism—it's fair, it's equal and it doesn't work for everyone. Many women in particular need to concentrate in order to achieve orgasm. When they have to give as well as receive pleasure, it can be distracting and make it more difficult to come.

Of course, there are exceptions. Some easily-orgasmic women like the distraction of sixty-nine because it enables them to stay in a state of high arousal for a longer period of time. That said, if mutual oral pleasuring doesn't really work for you, it's not because you're doing something wrong. It's simply not a great technique for some people.

Oral Sex and Power Play

If you want to bring some kinkiness into your erotic adventures, oral sex can be a fabulous way to play.

Either the receiver or giver can be dominant. If the receiver is the top (dominant), they can be very specific and directive about how they want to be pleasured. The tone can be kind or critical, depending on what dynamic works for both partners. The giver can be in bondage or required to submit in other ways, for instance by being instructed to not move and maintain a given position for a period of time. Or, the receiver can have their way with the giver's mouth and simply take their pleasure.

When the receiver is in the submissive role, the giver can bring their partner to the brink of orgasm and then stop, sip a drink, and begin again when they feel inclined or upon a proper request (or beg) from their bottom (submissive). They can restrain their partner physically, command them not to move, or tell them to order take-out over the phone without revealing to the person on the other end of the line exactly what is happening to their nether regions.

All power play is negotiated. Anything you do must have previously been consented to. If you're "making' your submissive wait to have an orgasm, you're not really making him or her do anything at all. You're playing pretend, the same way you played pretend as a child, only this time your genitals are involved. The moment you actually make someone do something against their will, then what you're doing is non-consensual, unethical and illegal—and no longer a game.

Penis-Specific Techniques

The biggest mistake people make when orally pleasuring a penis is starting with the familiar vigorous up-and-down bobbing motion. Since you're just getting going, it may be a while before the receiver is ready to orgasm—especially if he's not 16—which means that by the time he's ready to climax, you're bored and tired and your jaw is sore. Instead, start with gentler, teasing techniques and save your high-intensity moves for when he's getting close. You'll enjoy it a lot more and so will he!

A lot of men get really turned on when you make eye contact with them while their penis is near or in their mouth. Your look can be dominating, submissive, playful, sassy or tender—it's all good. (Sexy, too.) You're in charge here because you're in control of his orgasm, so claim your power with your gaze. For many guys, it's also a turn-on to see your mouth and tongue in action on his member. If you position yourself so he can see you and you can also look into his eyes, this will intensify his pleasure.

Here's another tip: Use more than your mouth. Give your mouth a hand—or two! Since your hands are much more versatile and stronger than your mouth, he will get a lot more stimulation and you'll have less strain on your jaw. Your hand also can be the gatekeeper as to how deeply he goes into your mouth—this will keep you from gagging. And use your breasts, women! For many guys, it's a total turn-on to see their cock plunge between a woman's breasts regardless of their size. This gives your mouth a break and it also opens the door to a great tease—you can breast-fuck him while your mouth sits perched barely beyond each stroke, a titillating possibility just out of reach.

Use lube generously. Your saliva dries out quickly. To give him even more pleasure, you want to be able to add some pressure and slide comfortably up and down, thus making lube your (and his) best friend. Options include:

- Silicone lube, which is long-lasting and tasteless.
- Water-based lubes, which come in a variety of textures, thicknesses, tastes and 'lastingness.'
- Flavored lubes, which can enhance how he tastes, but usually dry out quickly and get sticky.
- Coconut oil, an effective, tasty and fabulous alternative. Oil degrades latex condoms, though, so avoid it if condoms are part of the party.

Test out a few options at a local sex shop—they usually have sample bottles you can try by feeding a drop into your hand, then choosing what works best for you in terms of taste, texture and lastingness.

Here, again, porn is a bad teacher. On the Internet, you rarely see lube being applied to a cock. The usual moisturizer is spit, which isn't much use as a lube—it's used in porn because it comes across as raunchy and 'dirty.' If that turns you on or you are in a pinch without supplies, go for it. But it's not an effective, long-lasting way to lubricate a penis.

Three Keys to Great Fellatio

Show genuine enthusiasm, make eye contact, and use more than your mouth.

The Fine Art of Deep-Throating

No how-to on fellatio would be complete these days without a discussion of deep-throating. Three decades ago, when Linda Lovelace brought attention to this technique in the now-legendary movie *Deep Throat*, it was a novelty item. Now it's basically mandatory for mainstream porn actresses.

While being deep-throated certainly feels good, the turn-on is more psychological than physical. One reason: It's both dominant and submissive—dominant because of its python-like voraciousness, and submissive because the giver is basically saying, "Here I am, committing a literally unnatural act, overriding my gag reflex just to please you." It also offers up a great visual—"Wow, look at it go all the way in!" This is a great trifecta—but the turn-on is mostly in the guy's mind. If you just want to deliver physical pleasure, you'll often do better by using the hand and mouth techniques described here.

For those who wish to learn how to take a penis into your throat, here are a few tips.

Straighten out your neck and mouth (as though you are looking way up) so the penis you're pleasuring can travel on a straight line from lips to throat. Otherwise, it will need to bend to make the transition from mouth to throat and while the occasional dogleg penis is out there, most cocks are fairly straight and prefer to stay that way. (I'm referring to angle, not orientation.) One relatively easy way to align yourself for deep throat is to lie on your back with your neck and mouth hanging right at (not off) the edge of the bed.

The gag reflex is at the top back part of your mouth. When the tip of the penis (or anything) hits this area, we reflexively try to push it out—it's Mother Nature's way to keep us from choking. To keep from gagging, we need to:

- Angle the natural curve of the penis so it's aimed downwards, not up. This way the tip hits the bottom of the oral canal rather than the top where the gag reflex is located.

- Train the reflex to be less sensitive by practicing with a dildo or firm cucumber. Hold it against the area for 10 seconds at a time, a few times a day. The more you do this, the more control you'll have over your gag reflex and the better you'll be able to slide a large object—like, say, a penis—down your throat without your gag reflex protesting.

- Make sure you use lots of lubricant on the penis. You don't want something dry tickling the back of your throat. It doesn't feel good.

Last but not least, relax. If you're feeling anxious or tense, you probably won't be able to take him down very far. Try not to pressure yourself to learn it quickly or to do it every time with ease. Remember that you want to have fun, too. The more you enjoy taking his penis into your mouth or throat, the more he'll be delighted, too.

Fellatio-Specific Techniques

Breasts. Anything you can think of is good! Use the entire breast along the head and shaft. You can also stimulate the frenulum with your nipple or place the penis in your cleavage. These moves will be appreciated no matter how big or small your breasts are.

Food Play. Dribble honey, Bailey's Irish Cream, chocolate or a food of your choice on his cock. Then lick or nibble it off with appropriate sounds of gustatory and erotic appreciation.

Ice-Cream Cone Licks. Do long, teasing licks from bottom to top of penis (or from inner thigh up the penis to the nipple) with lots of eye contact. Because the sensitivity increases as you get closer to the head, tease him a little by stopping before the head once or twice. Then give a little extra tongue attention to the frenulum for the next lick.

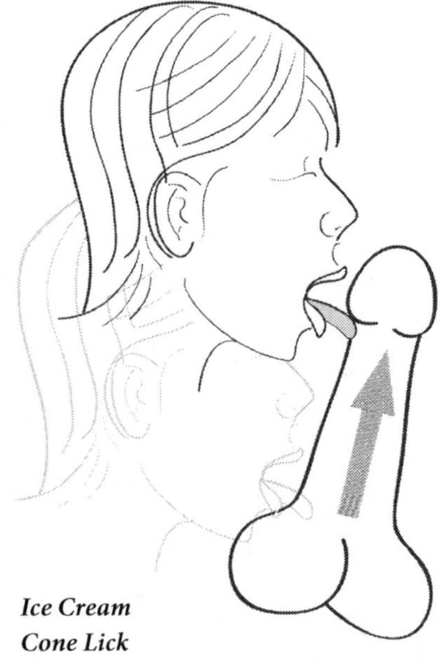

Ice Cream Cone Lick

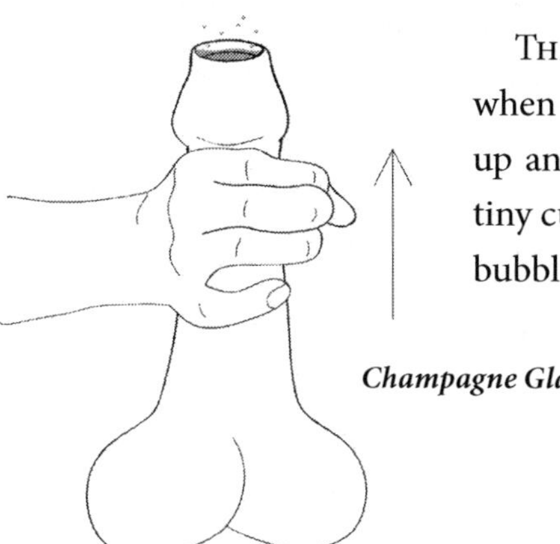

The Champagne Glass. If he's uncut, when he's not (very) aroused, pull his foreskin up and over the head of his penis to make a tiny cup. Pour a fizzy drink into it and sip. The bubbles deliver a super-tingly sensation.

Champagne Glass

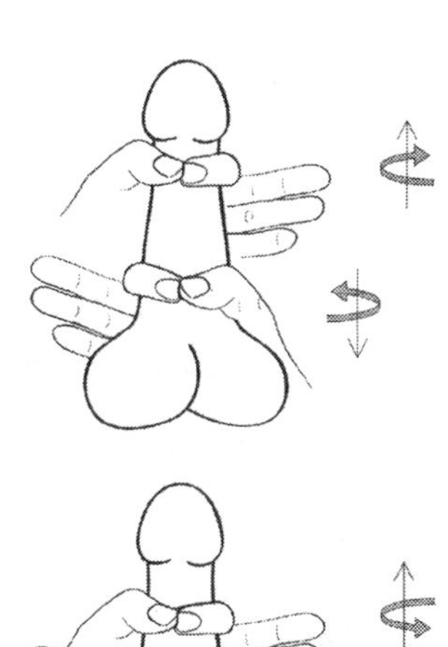

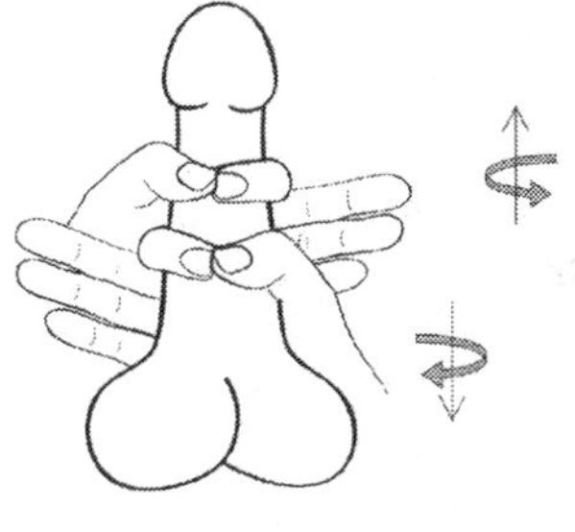

O-Ring. Make the 'okay' sign with both hands, slide them over the penis and slide your hands up and down in opposite directions. If you tend to get a sore jaw, you can use this move to counteract it. Keep the O-ring up against your mouth and notice that your hand naturally maintains the pressure while your jaw relaxes. Your mouth provides slipperiness and warmth while your hands offer the pressure—a decadent and delicious combination.

O-Ring

Opposites. Put one hand on the penis, gripping it in the middle. Put your mouth over the head and meet your lips with the thumb and index finger of your hand. Then move them in opposite directions, with the hand going down the shaft while the mouth goes up to the tip and then both returning to the midpoint again.

Opposites

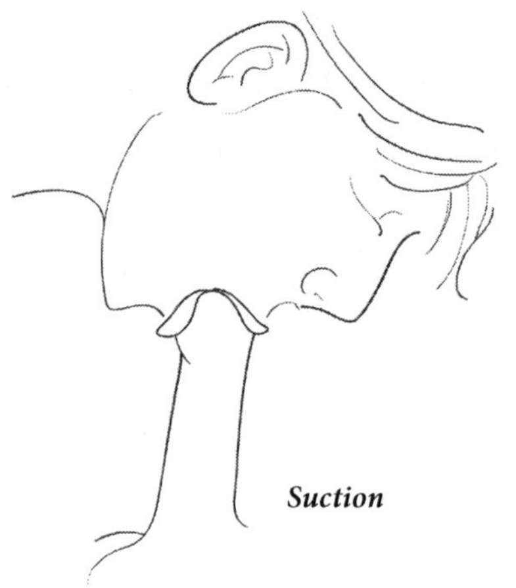

Suction

Suction. Feels fabulous just about anywhere. Here are two variations: 1) On the head of the penis, add a twist of your mouth as you suck there, or 2) suck on the frenulum or coronal ridge.

Tapping. Slap his penis against your pursed lips or your hand. This can help him get hard and feels great.

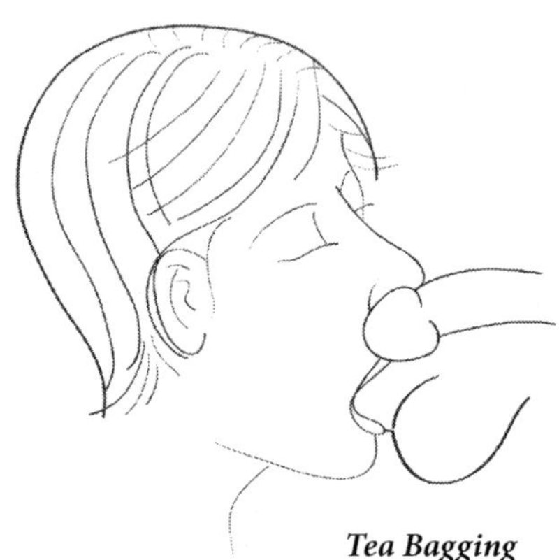

Tea Bagging

Tea Bagging. Suck on one testicle, pulling it into your mouth, then swirl your tongue around it and push it out gently.

Temperature Play. Use a warming or cooling lubricant, mints or lozenges—but only one or two!

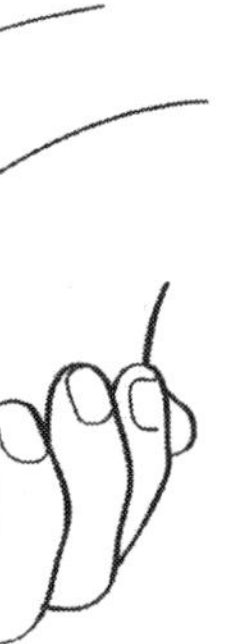

Meditation

Testicle Meditation. Hold the testicles gently in your hands and massage them sweetly like meditation balls.

Testicle Tease. Lick, flick, suck and roll the testicles with your tongue. (Be extra careful to not squeeze or otherwise be rough with them or he will be very unhappy and likely never let you near them again!)

The Dolphin. Your head tilts down with the top of your mouth leading with more pressure. On the way back up, the head tilts up with pressure more on the tongue. This slow deep movement makes your head look like a dolphin bobbing through the water.

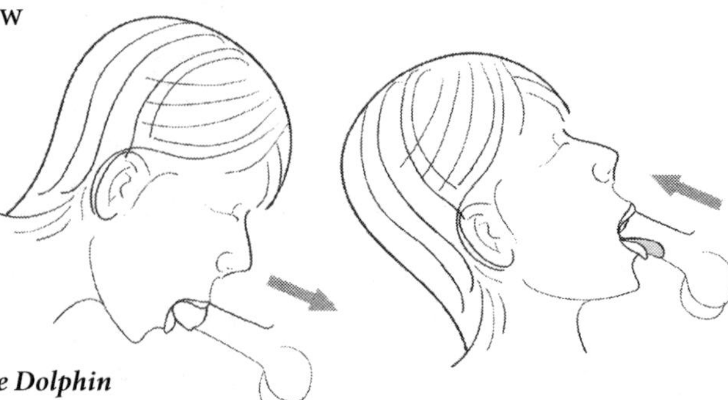

The Dolphin

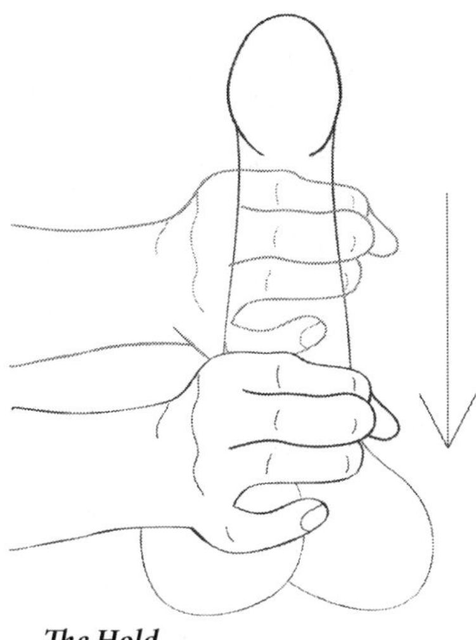

The Hold

The Hold. Pull down with a firm grip from midway on the shaft to the base, then hold and squeeze at the base. This makes the skin taut over the whole penis and heightens the sensations you create with your other hand and mouth.

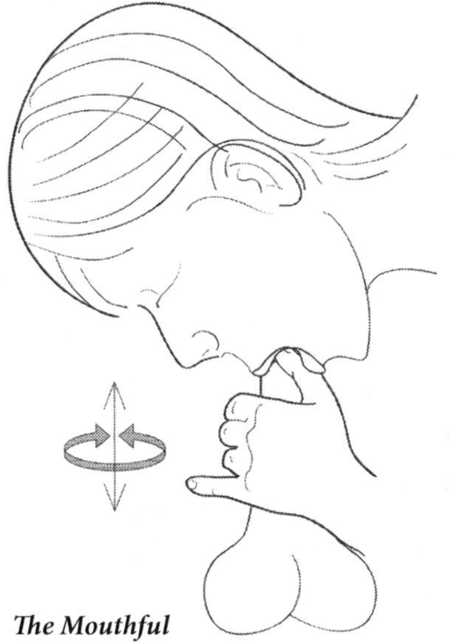

The Mouthful

The Mouthful. Position yourself at his side. Grab his shaft with your opposite hand (i.e., if he is on your left, use your right hand and vice versa) so that your palm is on the underside and your thumb is sticking up. Rub your thumb like a windshield wiper against his frenulum while the rest of your hand massages the shaft. Put your mouth over your thumb and penis, and bob up and down. Your thumb should be in the side of your mouth.

The Pigeon. Begin with your tongue under the shaft and your mouth at the tip. The tongue then pulls in and goes over the head and out over the top of the penis (so he is under your tongue), while the mouth goes down the shaft. Then pull him out of your mouth while your tongue comes back in over top of the head and slides back down the underside of the shaft. Your tongue should be going from the frenulum in a straight line over the top of the penis and then stimulating the head down towards the coronal ridge with the underside of your tongue. Start slowly.

The Pigeon

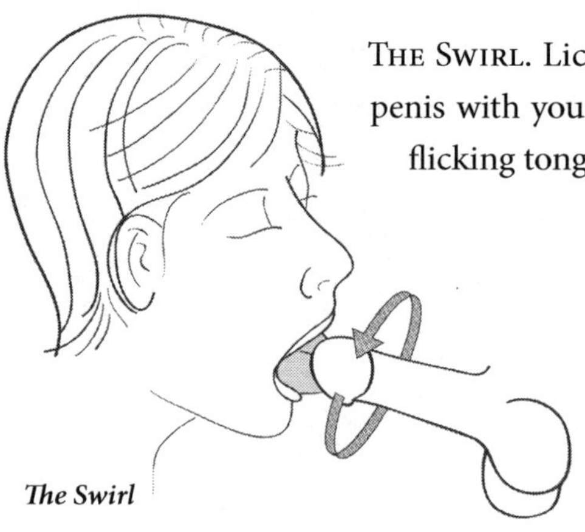

The Swirl

The Swirl. Lick in circles around the head of his penis with your mouth open or closed, or with a flicking tongue all the way around.

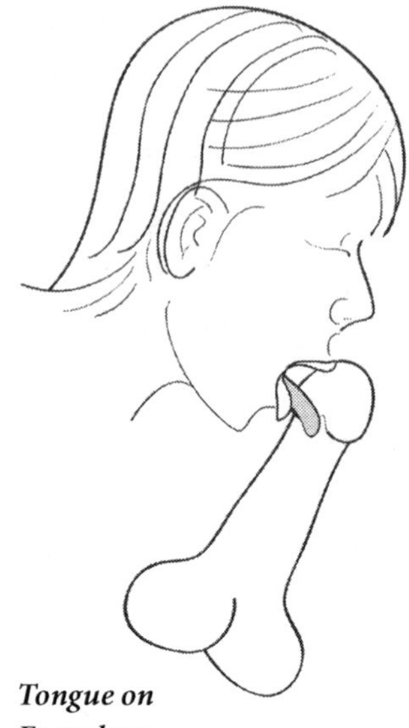

Tongue on Frenulum

Tongue on Frenulum. Any which way your tongue can contort will feel great—a soft, lazy tongue, a hard pointy tongue, a flicking tongue. Or, lick with your tongue out followed by a suck as though you were licking and then sucking on one of his lips.

Vibration. Use a vibrator along his shaft, against his perineum or testicles, or put it against your cheek while your mouth is on his sensitive areas to give him that extra buzz.

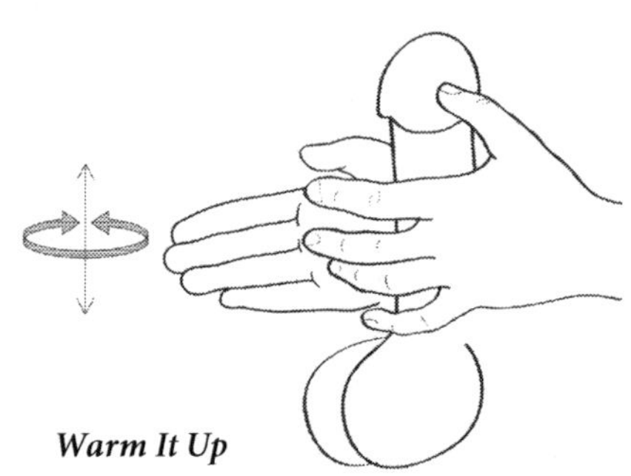

Warm It Up

Warm It Up. Make your hands flat and rub them back and forth over the shaft on the sides or back and front as though you were starting a fire. Do a gradual up-and-down motion as you press back and forth, preferably with your hands running over the frenulum on some strokes.

Wringing the Shaft. Use one or both hands as if you were wringing a towel, while your mouth works in tandem or focuses on the frenulum, head or testicles.

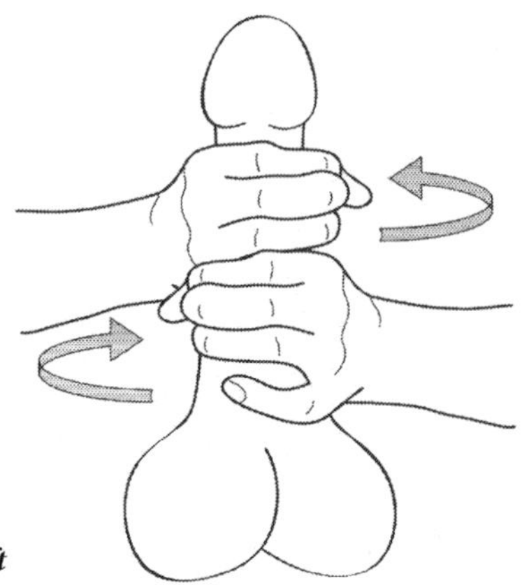

Wringing the Shaft

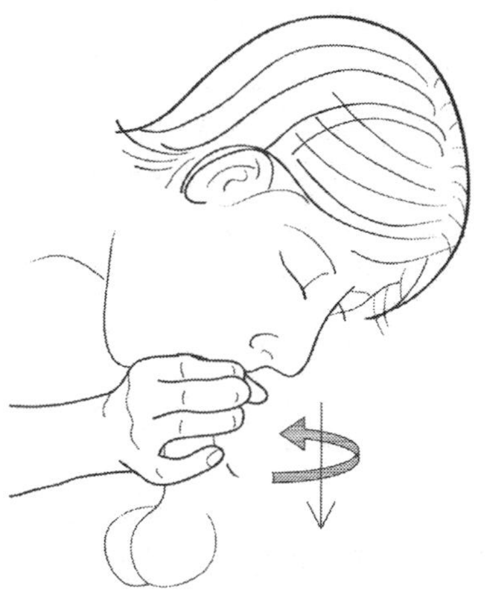

The Corkscrew. Similar to Wringing the Shaft, but both hand and mouth are connected and work as a single unit as you bob up and down with a slight twist side-to-side. (This is the one you want to save for the end to bring him over the edge).

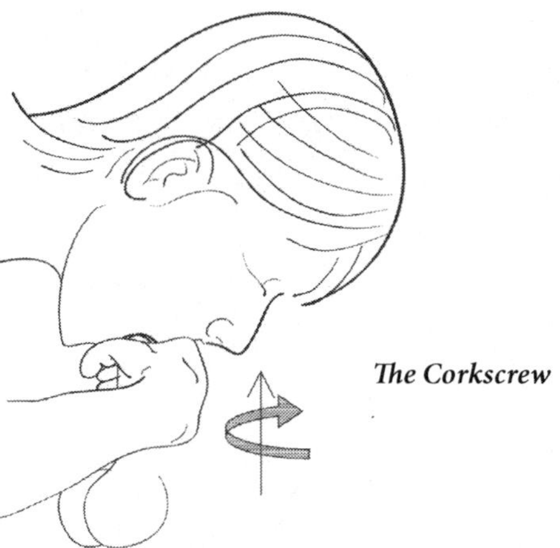

The Corkscrew

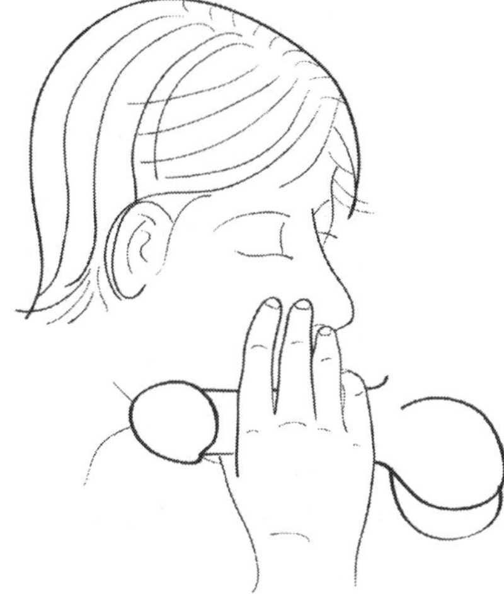

Dynamic Duo. If he needs a particular pressure and rhythm that you can't quite get, he can use his own hand on the shaft of his penis while you place your mouth on the head, the frenulum, his testicles, or anywhere that works in tandem with his hand.

The Harmonica

The Harmonica. If you don't like to swallow, this one is a gem. When he is close to coming, place yourself to the side of his penis and put your wide open mouth on one side with full contact between your lips and his penis. Put your hand on the opposite side of his penis. Either he moves and you hold still or you move your mouth and hand together up and down the shaft as though you were playing the harmonica. The intensity can be enough for him to ejaculate and it won't go into your mouth!

Vulva-Specific Techniques

The #1 request women make is to slow down.

And then, when you think you've slowed down enough, slow down some more. See if you can trace your tongue gently from the bottom to the top of her labia in no less than 15 seconds.

(Yes, that slowly.)

Women are often slower to reach orgasm than men and many need to be emotionally relaxed and not distracted in order to come. We frequently feel rushed or guilty if we take 'too long.' The slower you go, the more you communicate you aren't in a hurry, and this makes it easier for her to relax.

When you find something that works, don't stop or change unless she asks you to. Most women need a consistent rhythm in order to orgasm, so you will need to maintain a constant pace to take her over the edge. Don't rush, and don't treat her vulva like a buffet either, where you try a bit of this and then a bit of that. If you try too many techniques, and if they're done in a way that feels incoherent, it will be hard for her to surrender to the sensations and relax fully into the pleasure of what you're doing. If you're doing Technique A—like, say, slowly licking her labia—keep doing it for at least a minute so she can get used to the sensation. (Unless, of course, she specifically asks you to stop.)

How do you know when to stop and when to keep going? She'll give the cues. If she moans or offers her vulva up for more, it's a pretty good sign you're doing something right. If she's mute and motionless, it might mean you should try something else. Don't move on, though, until you've given the move enough time for her to start showing interest—the one-minute rule still applies. There's a delicate balance here—her silence may mean her arousal is building, and it may mean she's wondering what's for dinner. If you're not sure, stick up your head and ask.

If you're lucky enough to be the person who's got someone's head between your thighs, there's a lesson in this for you, too. Receive actively. Let them know if something's working for you and also, clearly and kindly, if it's not. That person's face is there for your ecstasy. Don't be shy about taking charge and steering it to your destination. You can even ask your partner to stay in one place while you move your pelvis to get the right pressure, speed and technique.

The clitoral tip is a fabulous erogenous zone, but don't go there directly. For one thing, it's incredibly sensitive. Many women can't abide having it touched until they're quite aroused, while other women don't want it to be touched directly, ever. Also, women have an entire erectile network in their vulva (see Sheri Winston's chapter on genital anatomy and sexuality). The clitoral tip is far from the only game in town. The inner and outer labia (lips) are great places to stimulate, as are the zones just outside the labia, which respond positively to firm pressure from a well-lubed finger or your tongue (which just happens to come pre-lubed). There's also the clitoral shaft, covered by the hood, directly above the clitoral tip.* The more you play with her whole erectile network, the more aroused she will get and the more spectacular her orgasms will be. And that's why you're down there, right?

While it's natural to be clit-centric, she'll probably appreciate it if you're not, especially at first. This isn't only a matter of spending quality time with the rest of her vulva. You might also want to take time off to nibble and kiss the insides of her thighs or curve of her belly, or to run your hands up her torso and down her legs. This spreads the energy, slows things down and deepens her arousal so that when she comes, it'll be especially spectacular.

Three Keys to Great Cunnilingus

Slow down, don't be clit-centric, and slow down some more.

Hands and toys are also useful in tandem with your tongue. Make sure that your fingers or toys are well-lubricated when you use them on her vulva or inside her vagina. There is no natural lubrication on the outside, and the inside can produce varying quantities of lubrication. If she is not naturally wet inside the vagina, don't take it as an insult. Some women lubricate a lot, others not so much—and different factors such as medications, relaxation, water or alcohol in her system, or monthly cycle can affect her wetness. Any commentary on her perceived arousal can make her dry up even more from worry about her body's performance. Just add some lube and carry on with giving her pleasure.

Teasing is a fine thing so long as you don't bring her arousal down too much. Again, it's a delicate balance. Make her hungry (or, even better, desperate) to have your mouth and tongue back on her vulva again.

So: Take it slowly and gently. Do no clit-licking before its time. Wait for cues from her, verbal or non-verbal, to know the moment has arrived. Again—and I know I'm reprising a familiar theme here—a great way to find out is to ask. Don't beat around the bush, so to speak. Ask directly: "Would you like me to lick your clit now?" If she grunts, that probably means yes. Ditto if she thrusts her crotch in your face so hard you can't breathe.

* What's commonly called the clitoris is really the clitoral tip—the clitoris is a much more extensive structure.

Specific Cunnilingus Techniques

Grazing. Super-gentle, slow tongue along the labia. Take 15 seconds to graze from below the opening to the vagina to the top of the clitoris.

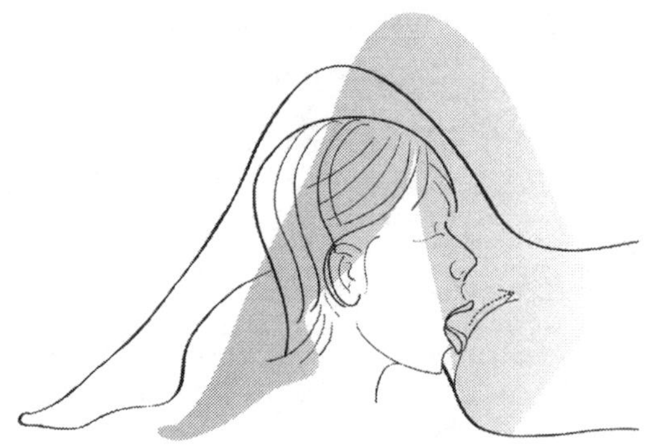

Grazing

Tongue Roll. Just like you learned in grade school—cup the underside of the clitoris with your rolled tongue.

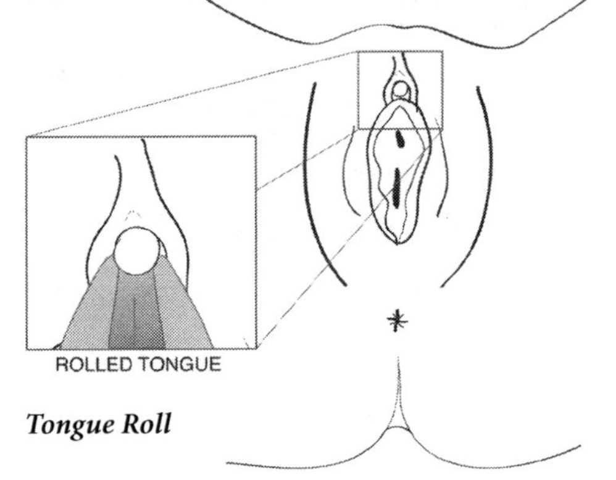

Tongue Roll

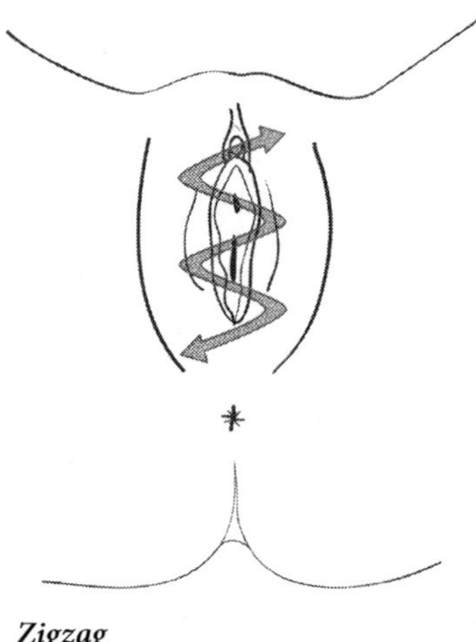

Zigzag

Zigzag. Gently and slowly move your tongue up and down across the whole vulva in a zigzag motion.

Hard Ice Cream. Lick firmly and slowly between the inner and outer labia. This reaches the erectile tissue that's under the surface and forms part of the clitoris. Pretend you have two tongues: your actual one on one side of the labia and a well-lubed finger on the other.

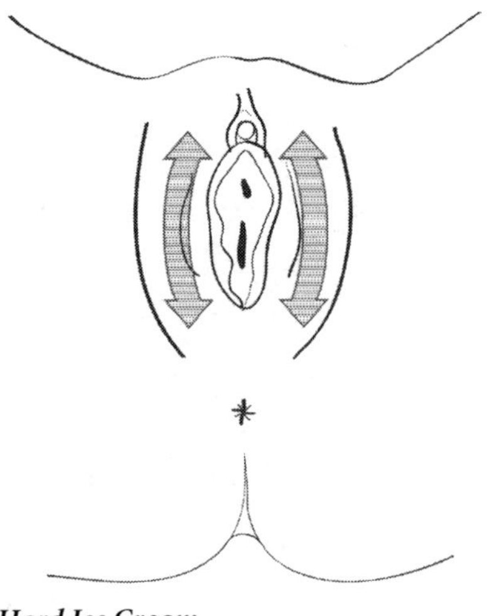

Hard Ice Cream

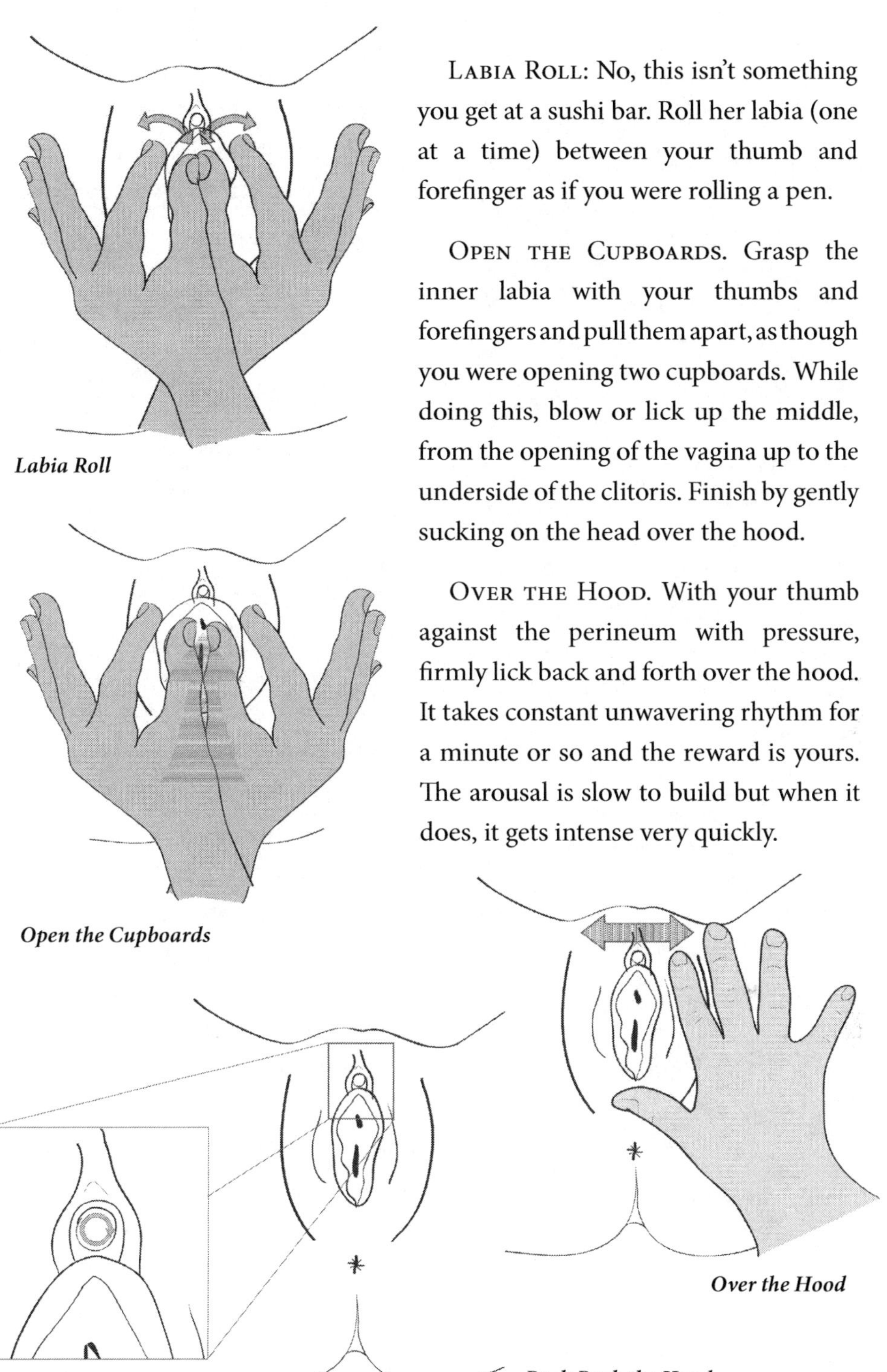

Labia Roll

Open the Cupboards

Over the Hood

Push Back the Hood

Labia Roll: No, this isn't something you get at a sushi bar. Roll her labia (one at a time) between your thumb and forefinger as if you were rolling a pen.

Open the Cupboards. Grasp the inner labia with your thumbs and forefingers and pull them apart, as though you were opening two cupboards. While doing this, blow or lick up the middle, from the opening of the vagina up to the underside of the clitoris. Finish by gently sucking on the head over the hood.

Over the Hood. With your thumb against the perineum with pressure, firmly lick back and forth over the hood. It takes constant unwavering rhythm for a minute or so and the reward is yours. The arousal is slow to build but when it does, it gets intense very quickly.

Push Back the Hood. Use your lips to pull back the hood and expose the head of clit. Then run circles with your tongue around the head of the clit. Do this very slowly and gently, with each cycle lasting one to five seconds. If you go slowly and gently enough, even the most sensitive clitorises can often enjoy the ecstasy.

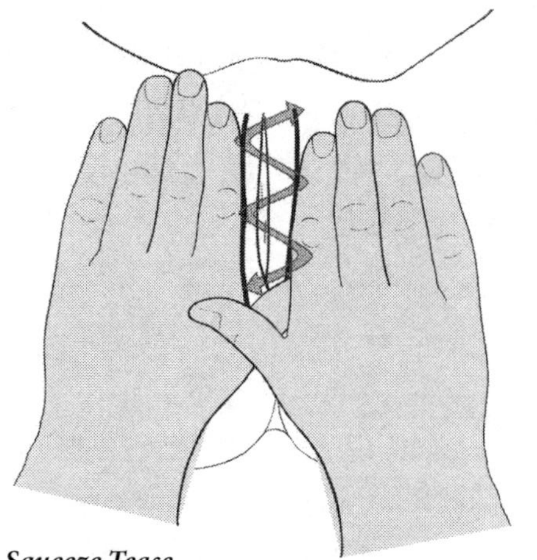

Squeeze Tease: With two hands, squeeze all the folds of her inner and outer labia together into the middle, then move your hands up and down in opposite directions.

Squeeze Tease

Squeeze Shaft of the Clit: Grab onto the shaft of the clitoris (over the hood) and move up and down with firm pressure if she likes. Some call this a 'clit hand job.'

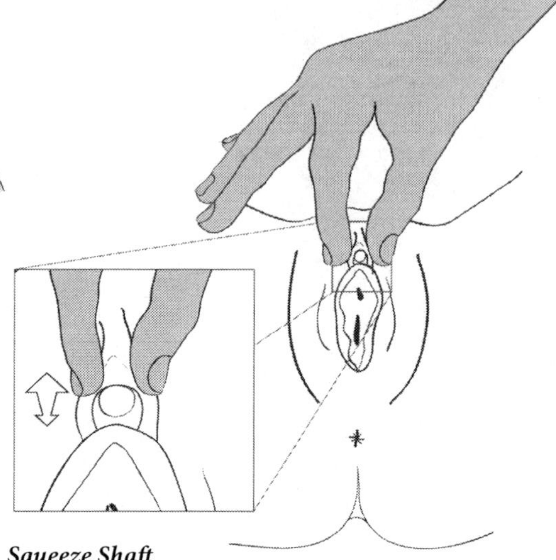

Squeeze Shaft

Sucking on Tip of the Clit. Pull down on the entire clitoral area, sucking on the hood over the clitoris with a flicking tongue or just pressure.

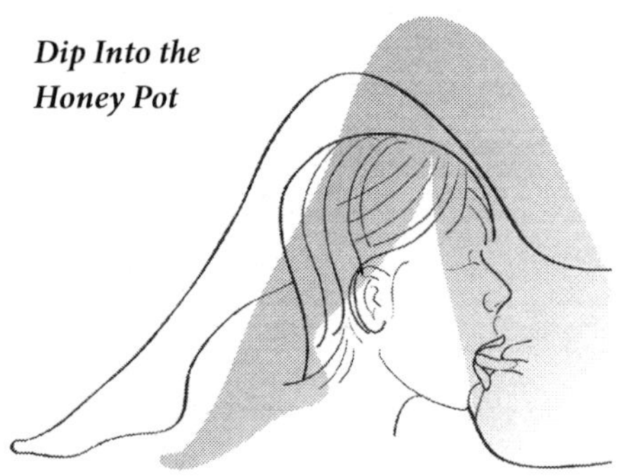

Dip Into the Honey Pot

Dip Into the Honey Pot. Insert your tongue into the entrance of the vagina. You can dart in and out or go slowly with large circles at the opening. You can also roll your tongue. Many women say the most enjoyable part of penetration is when they're first entered, so why not spend a lot of time there?

Figure-8. Circle around the clitoris and then cross over and down around the vagina and across the perineum and back up again in a figure-eight pattern. This technique connects the clitoris with the vaginal area.

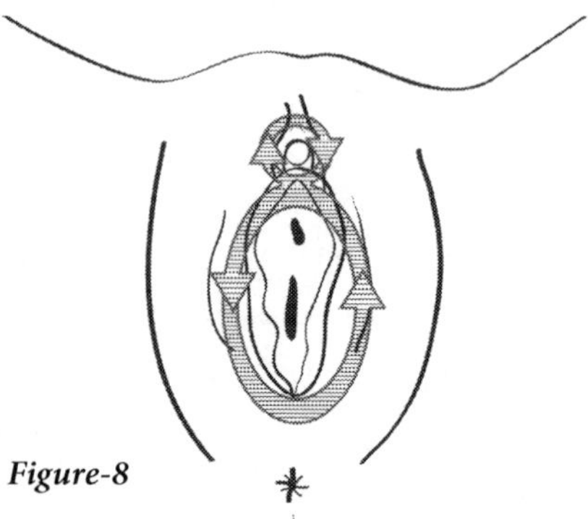

Figure-8

G-Spotting (Double Your Pleasure). Insert two fingers or a toy to contact the specific place on the roof of her vagina where she likes it—it can be anywhere from one knuckle in to the depth of a whole finger. Many receivers like the 'come here' motion, but the peace sign (separating two fingers) and the windshield wiper (back and forth together) work better for some.

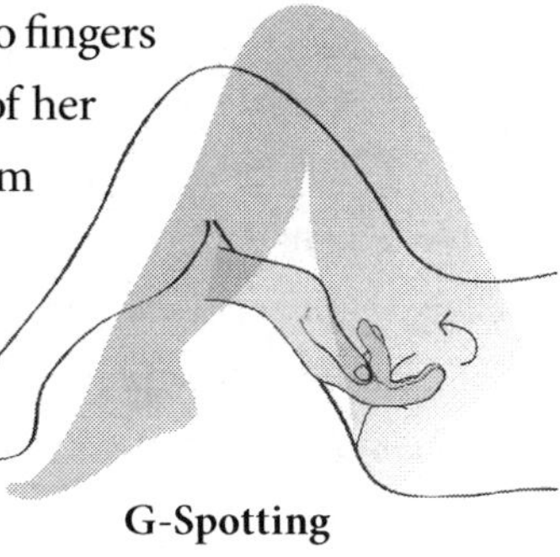

G-Spotting

* * *

Here's an extra-credit move if you're in a long-term relationship with the person you're going down on. Learn the vocabulary in these sidebars or invent your own shared language. If you're craving a certain move, it's great to be able to ask for it with a simple word or two. When you're in the throes of ecstasy, it interrupts the flow to say, "You know that move you do when you're licking my lips really slowly and you use a butterfly motion? Would you try that, please?" And then they don't quite get it, and by the time you've muddled through, you've got to re-group and more or less start over.

This is not where you want to be going. Shorthand is a fine thing.

And so is a slow tongue, and, let's not stop there, the entire gourmet treat of oral pleasure.

This concludes my oral presentation. Take from it what you will and enjoy!

SEXY SUMMARY

Oral sex has lots of negative stories associated with it. It may be necessary for you to clear them out in order to fully enjoy the pleasures of fellatio and/or cunnilingus.

Givers, enthusiasm matters. The more you express your pleasure, the more you'll please.

Communication matters, too. A lot. Don't be shy about asking for what you want! A shorthand language can help a lot here.

Sixty-nine isn't for everyone. If it doesn't work for you, you're not alone.

Don't copy mainstream porn. It's a bad model. Be in the moment. Discover what works for you and your partner.

Oral sex is a wonderful treat. And: Nothing requires you to do it.

JON PRESSICK *is the sexual community's gadabout. He's a writer, editor, broadcaster, pundit, organizer and provocateur. Jon recently wrapped up work on his first edition as editor of the long-running book series Best Sex Writing 2015, due out in early 2015. Jon also contributes a bi-weekly column "Sex Stories We Love" for Kinkly.com. You can find his writing daily at Sex in Words.*

When not writing about sex, Jon talks about sex as one of the co-hosts of Sex City. He's also a frequent guest on numerous other podcasts. If you happen to be in Toronto, you may have seen Jon strip in a burlesque show, talk on a panel at a sex conference, read his Choose Your Own Sex Adventure *erotica or lead a workshop on prostate pleasure.*

Jon can be reached at jon.pressick@gmail.com.

CHAPTER THREE

Anal Sex

by Jon Pressick

The biggest question people have about anal sex isn't about 'how,' 'when' or 'with whom.' It is 'why?' Specifically—"Why would *anyone* want to be on the receiving end of anal sex?" Their concerns run the gamut from possible physical pain and discomfort to social stigma.

As someone who writes about sex and has a special fondness for ass play, I have two different answers when people inquire about anal. My official explanation is that it is a pleasurable experience, it can create special bonds between the partners, and it can also have health benefits.

My unofficial answer is, "Because anal sex rocks!"

I am an enthusiastic ambassador of all things ass. When people object that "Anal is dirty," I say, "In all the best ways!" When people say, "Anal will hurt," I say, "Not if you do it right!" And when people say, "Anal is unnatural," I suggest they put down their smartphones, get out of their cars, spread their cheeks and get down to business with one of the simplest, most natural pleasures this green Earth has to offer.

Anal Pleasure Options

There are many delightful options for awesome ass action. Whether you're into sweet and gentle or hard and wild, anal comes in every shade of sexy.

First, a quick note on terminology. Throughout the chapter I will refer to 'pitcher' and 'catcher.' This baseball-themed analogy refers to the person (the pitcher) who is touching, caressing, licking or penetrating the other person's (the catcher's) ass. Don't worry, no uniforms are required (unless you choose to wear them!).

Fingers. A little digital delight is the usual entry point for this less usual port of access. Ass fingering can be its own delight, or it can be used during oral sex, intercourse or any other time you think it might work.

Oral. Oral-anal contact, also called rimming, is a sensuous encounter like no other. Using your lips and tongue on someone's ass is perhaps the most intimate experience two people can share. Because of the fears of mess and the need for proper hygiene, prior communication and consent is a must—in fact, this goes for all things anal. Whether it is light little kisses or getting your tongue a couple inches in there, make sure you're both very comfortable with what will be happening. You may or may not want to pursue barrier options when pursuing rimming.

Toys. There is a tremendous selection of toys on the market these days for both male and female asses. It just might be the largest growth area in the sex toy industry. Butt plugs, vibrators, prostate massagers, lubes—there's a bounty of booty booty out there! Because women's and men's anal areas differ, there are toys that are specific to each gender. There are also plenty that work for any ass.

Men, don't feel barred from using female sex toys, and vice-versa. Find out what works for you. But don't take that mix and match too far. Sex toys should never travel between different orifices without being thoroughly cleaned along the way.

Penile Penetration. When people think of anal sex, this is what usually comes to mind. The popular perception is that anal is all about cock in ass, be it in a heterosexual or homosexual context. But as this list shows, there are many other options.

Pegging. This involves the use of a strap-on dildo by a woman on a man.* For many years, this activity was rarely spoken of. The groundbreaking instructional porn film *Bend Over Boyfriend* changed this and launched a shift in awareness and attitude that has resulted in more and more men getting turned on at the prospect of taking it in the ass. The question of "Does this make me gay?" still hangs heavy over many men and we'll address that later on.

*** A bit of etymology: The term 'pegging' came from an invitation by sex columnist Dan Savage to his readers to come up with a term for "woman pitching, man catching' anal dildo play. It is not used for woman-on-woman or man-on-man anal dildo play. I'm unaware of any term for these activities.**

Fisting. With fisting, you're entering advanced ass-sex territory. It's just what it sounds like—the same as vaginal fisting, only in another (and less elastic) orifice.

Fisting is a long, involved and—if you're into it—entirely amazing experience. As with all anal acts, lube is essential, but it isn't the most important ingredient. That would be patience. I mean, think about it. Can a hand go up someone's butt quickly and easily? It will probably take multiple sessions to achieve the Promised Hand. Whether vaginal or anal, fisting is a new physical process for your body to learn. As your partner slowly moves more and more of their hand into you, your body needs to learn to accommodate that presence. You might possibly take someone's whole hand on the first go, but it's more likely that your body will need to learn to accommodate something that sizable. Some people may never be able to take a whole hand. It all depends on your anatomy and the size of the hand.

Even if you can't take in a whole hand, you can still enjoy partial fisting. Most of the enjoyment of fisting comes from the pressure exerted on your body as the fingers and hand go in. That sensation is electric! As more hand is pushed into you, more sensations explode across your body. This can make you wild, even if it's not the entire hand you're taking in.

Go with your comfort level in considering these options. Whatever works for you—and doesn't work for you—is okay.

The Power of Solo Play

I strongly recommend solo play as a path to anal self-discovery. Find out for yourself what feels good and what doesn't. How slow do you have to go, and what moves work best, for you to take an object up your rectum without pain? What size feels best to you? How about prostate massage (if you're a guy)? The more you know about what you like and don't, the better you'll be able to guide your partner.

The first time you put something in your ass, your response may not be entirely positive. It can feel, well, *unnatural*—nature designed the anus to be an exit ramp, after all, not an entryway. Your ass is working in reverse and may be as confused about its feelings as you are. You may experience the sensation as an odd and not pleasing sense of fullness and constriction. If you start off with something small, it's likelier to feel good, and if you wait till you're aroused before sticking something in your bum, that will serve you well, too.

If ass play is in your future, that initial confusing sensation will start feeling good—rich with the promise of pleasures to come. Over time, if you become an ass aficionado, any early anxiety will go away and you'll open to the amazing pleasure anal sex can deliver.

And if you decide that ass play isn't in your future, that's fine too.

As you play with your own ass, discovering what you do and do not like, make sure you take some mental notes that you can apply when you try this with a partner. (And, yes, you can be as anal as you want in your note-taking!)

Anal Anxieties

People have three main fears when considering anal sex: mess, pain and stigma. These are all legitimate concerns, and they also all have good answers. We'll touch on stigma later. For now, let's look at the fear of mess and the fear of pain.

Others may disagree, but I'm convinced that the phrase "shit happens" originated with a messy anal sex encounter. I'm not sure who uttered it, the pitcher or the catcher, but I hope it was uttered in an appropriate spirit of acceptance.

When you're playing with someone's rectum, given its primary anatomical function, it's always possible that fecal matter will come into the equation. Indeed, if you become a regular at this activity, at some point it *will* happen. With proper communication and preparation, though, the potential for an unpleasant encounter with someone's eliminations can be pretty much, er, eliminated.

The chances of encountering a full bowel movement are miniscule. To understand why this is so, let's briefly review anal anatomy:

- The *anus*, known colloquially as the asshole, is the ass's entry (and exit) point. It's closed pretty tight as a matter of course—you don't want stuff leaking out, after all.

- Surrounding the anus is a circular rim of slightly raised muscles. These are the *anal sphincters*, a pair of circular muscles, one inner and one outer, that act like a drawstring to keep the rectal pouch closed. Their main job is to keep feces from spilling out of the rectum.

- The *anal canal* is the short passage—about one inch long—that separates the rectum from the anus. It's encircled by the anal sphincters. It feels like what it is, a gateway into something bigger.

- The *rectum* is the last anatomic segment of the large intestine before the anus. It's about five inches long. If you put a toy or penis into the ass, the rectum is the part you're stimulating, along with the sphincters.

- The rectum is technically a continuation of the *sigmoid colon*, which is the last (and lowest) part of the large intestine. For practical purposes, we can differentiate between the intestines (the colon and above) and the ass (the rectum and below).

With this for background, let's return to the subject at hand—poop. Feces are stored in the sigmoid colon. The rectum is an exit ramp for excretory matter, not a parking garage. Elimination through the rectum only happens when the body sends the appropriate signals. Anal sex doesn't deliver these messages. You're not at risk of suddenly having a bowel movement if someone puts something up your ass.

However, as poop travels down the rectum on its way to the outside world, it's not uncommon for residual bits of fecal matter to be left behind in the rectum. Thus the risk isn't about suddenly having a big, stinking stool on your sheets, it's about possible dribs and drabs of brown stuff. Which, of course, isn't appetizing either.

Lifestyle plays a significant factor in determining poop potential. When the ass in question belongs to someone with a bad diet or digestive ailments, it may not be a fun playground, especially if you're easily grossed out. Even if you're a health nut and clean freak, one really great curry could make for a challenging anal-sex encounter.

If your or your partner's preference is to be squeaky-clean, you can prepare for anal sex with an enema. This practice is controversial. The main concern is that it can inflame the rectum's mucosal lining. With natural enemas like warm water, the risk is negligible, although if you overdo any enema, it can be a problem.

Personally, I'm not a big fan of enemas. I don't find them necessary. Pay attention to your body and you'll know if it's a good time for ass play.

Some people like to play erotically with enemas because they like the feeling of being filled up, of expelling liquid, or both. This certainly isn't everyone's cup of Fleet's, but if that's what you fancy, go for it.

I recommend having natural baby wipes nearby for quick and easy mess response along with a receptacle for anally-used toys and a garbage can for barriers that you're done with. The action is often still going hot and heavy when the time for ass play has ended. You don't want to have to brake for clean-up.

Now that we have cleaned up the fear of mess, let's turn to the fear of pain. It's true that anal sex can hurt, but then so can vaginal. With the proper care, attention, technique and focus, pain during anal sex is completely avoidable. Anytime anything goes into one of your orifices, it should feel good. Or great.

Or *amazing*. If pain occurs during anal sex, it can be due to factors like poor technique, lack of patience, lack of lube and the inability to relax.

You can overcome these challenges with care, experimentation and communication. And by going slowly.

Here's an important point to remember about pain. It's a subjective experience. The more aroused we are, the likelier we are to experience something as pleasurable, not painful. The nipple tweak that makes someone yelp with pain when not aroused may make them moan with pleasure once they're turned on and hot. Similarly with ass play—timing is everything.

However, if you try and try and anal touch just doesn't feel right to you, your body is probably telling you to move on to different pleasures. Some people just aren't anatomically built for these activities. If your body is saying no, be sure to listen to it. Fortunately, your body has countless other lovely parts to play with!

The best way to ensure a pain-free experience is by warming up the ass very slowly. Don't just go barging in—the ass is a receptive organ but it needs to be courted.

For many people, this starts with warming up the butt cheeks, starting laterally toward the hips. Stroke them in a steady circular motion and gradually narrow the arc until you're staying inside the ass crack, circling the anus. Don't go in yet!

Next, you'll want to tease the sphincters open. Begin with the external rim and circle it with a well-lubed, firm, non-tentative finger or pair of fingers. Maintain consistent pressure. Eventually the sphincter will start to relax and open up. It'll almost feel as if it's asking you to slip a finger inside. Do as requested, but don't plunge beyond the anal canal into the rectum yet. Rim the muscle wall with a slow, firm but not rough touch, or alternatively apply firm pressure to one area of the sphincter muscle until you feel it release, then move to another area. One option is to work your way around slowly, as if the wall were a clock face and you were pausing at each hour to gently but firmly apply pressure. Eventually the entire band of muscle will relax open and the top of your finger will be pulled in and through.

Even now, you don't want to hurry. Keep circling slowly and firmly. In the ass, every move is magnified, so use small, slow motions. Super-slow motions. Your fingers are in a dialogue with the rectum. If it's not opening, it's telling you it's not ready for deeper or more energetic penetration. If you feel it relaxing and opening, go ahead and slide in more deeply. Maybe try some very slow thrusting instead of circling motions and see how that's received.

Pitchers, it can be helpful to verbally remind your receiver to relax and let go. Sometimes all it takes to get the ass to open is a clear instruction to do so.

There's an art to receiving, too. Just because someone's doing you doesn't mean you're in a passive role. Receive actively. Feel free to clearly and politely tell your do-er what is and isn't working for you. Give specific guidance if you think it will help.

Other useful ways to support the process include consciously breathing slowly and deeply, relaxing the mouth and throat (which relaxes the muscles at the bottom of the pipe as well), making round-mouthed "Oh!" sounds, and imagining your ass releasing and opening.

If at any point there's the slightest bit of pain, ask the do-er to pause in their anal play and hold their fingers (or whatever) perfectly still. As the receiver, breathe deeply and consciously relax your inner ass muscles. When the cramp or twinge resolves, return to those super-slow movements. Stop the action as required to allow for relaxation.

Givers, be attuned to those signals. If your receptive partner says to freeze, respond immediately. You are gaining the ass's trust by never pushing beyond its pleasure.

All this can take two, five, ten minutes or more. Don't hurry—patience is one of the keys to great anal sex—and always—*always!*—use plenty of lube.

You'll know the ass wants more action when it, or its owner, is begging you for more.

Communicate, Communicate, Communicate

There are three 'communicates' in this header because anal play requires three types of communication.

The first is the standard, critically important, mandatory pre-sex play conversation—only this time it's about anal. You've just met someone and it's pretty clear there's a bedroom in your future. What sort of activities are you open to? What are you not open to? Are you receptive to anal penetration? If so, with what? Will you pitch but not catch? How about rimming? What are your safer sex requirements? Is there pegging in your future? These are the sort of things you want to get totally clear about before your clothes come off and the blood leaves your brain.

The second anal-sex discussion involves whether to have anal sex *today*. This conversation you'll have with someone who is already an anal-play partner. Are there reasons to not take the backdoor route, like maybe your recent bout of diarrhea? Just because you love anal sex doesn't mean you want to do it this evening. Even if that case of diarrhea isn't a stopper for you, it might be for your partner. You owe it to them to speak up—they have the right to choose how much potential mess they'll have to deal with.

A great place to have this conversation is a shared steamy, sexy shower as you're getting ready for sex. If anal sex turns out to be off the table for the evening, there are ways to provide consolation.

The third anal-sex conversation happens when you're actually playing anally. Clear, constructive feedback helps enormously. Don't be afraid to get creative and sexy! Clear and constructive doesn't have to sound like a manual. Slip those hot words and well-placed moans into your talk to heighten the mood.

I suppose it's theoretically possible to over-communicate about sex, but I have trouble imagining it. If you're going to err, do it on the side of excess. The importance of communication can't be overstated.

The Two Keys to Great Anal Sex

There are two key elements to having mind-blowing anal sex. One you buy at the store, the other you have to practice.

Once you decide to try anal sex, you'll want to be fully prepared. This means getting yourself a lube you love. This isn't to say that ass-fucking can't be done without lube, but it isn't advisable and it's potentially dangerous. Nobody wants rips or tears in their anus, so get out there and stock up!

Back in the day, before personal lubricants were a big industry, the go-to items to facilitate anal penetration were things like butter, margarine, Crisco and Vaseline. (There's a memorable line in the 1972 art-house classic *Last Tango in Paris* where Marlon Brando says to Maria Schneider, his young partner, "Get the butter.") In theory these all still work—after all, they're still slippery—but they are also oil-based and not good in the bum. They can leave a coating on the walls of the rectum that can contribute to bacterial and other infections. They are also a no-no if you're using a condom, as oil breaks down and weakens latex. Bye-bye, safer sex!

> *The two keys to great anal sex are lube and patience.*

Instead of these homemade make-do's, take a trip to your local pharmacy or sex shop to check out the wide assortment of lubes that are available. Many sex shops sell small trial sizes so you can figure out which is best for you. You'll probably want to try a whole selection because finding the lube you love is a lot like buying clothes: everyone has their own preference.

There are two types of recommended lube—water-based and silicone-based. Both have their pluses and minuses:

- Water-based lubes are slick and smooth. The problem with them is that they can dry out, which means that if you go for a marathon butt sex session, you can be left with a sticky residue. You can remedy this by applying more water-based lube or by spritzing the affected area with water, which will bring back the lube's initial slickness and smoothness.

- Silicone-based lubes are super-slick and meant to go that extra mile, again and again and again. Once you apply, you're good to go! (Or come.) They have a thinner texture than water-based and so they don't clean up as easily as their water-based counterparts. Give a good scrub afterwards or you just might be sliding out of your seat! The bigger downside is that you can't use silicone-based lube with silicone toys. It will destroy them.

Whichever lube you choose, remember that you can never have enough of it in, around and on an ass. Go wild! And keep the bottle nearby for handy reapplication.

The other key to great anal sex is patience. It's crucial to take things slow. Whether you're pitching or catching, slow down and show restraint. You're not in a race. Nor is there any particular benefit to penetrating or being penetrated in record time. The last time I checked, the Guinness Book of World Records didn't have a category for fastest ass penetration.

Warming up, ramping up and lubing up are three hot and sexy ways to practice that patience. Take a lot of time to play with other parts of the body before moving on to the ass. Massage is a great relaxer—so are orgasms! After you stimulate other erogenous parts of the body with your warm-up, move down to the anus. Whatever you're into, start out slow and increase your ministrations slowly and surely.

Earlier I gave specific guidance about this. The important thing to remember is to go really slowly until you're both absolutely, totally sure it'll feel great for you both if you don't hold back any longer. There's this place of comfort, energy and connection that you reach. Once you're there, you'll know what to do.

And, even then, err on the side of going slow.

Prostate Play and the Perineal Sponge

While everyone's anus is rich in delicate tissue and sensitive nerve endings, men and women have distinct playgrounds offering different exciting rides.

The prostate has become a unifying symbol of progressive men's sexuality. This walnut-sized gland, which can be felt through the front wall of the male rectum, is now a hotspot of fun and wild orgasms. Men who have discovered the erotic potential of their prostates sometimes refer to it as a revolutionary moment in their sex lives.

But just as anal sex itself is something you need to ease into, so is prostate massage. That first time you touch it with a finger, toy or cock, be ready to see your man nearly jump out of his skin. Prostate stimulation is unlike any other feeling in a man's body. It's intense! Go slowly. Take time and take breaks too if the sensations are too strong. You might want to pull away from the prostate or pull out altogether, whatever is best for him.

A great way to access the prostate is with a nicely lubed finger using that seductive 'come hither' motion. It is accessed through the front wall of the anal cavity, so you will have to adjust your hand position depending on whether he is on his back or on his hands and knees. If he is on his back, have your hand palm-up and curl that finger toward you. If he is on his knees, go palm-down and push your finger toward the floor. Keep it up and the experience will be mind-blowing—and potentially load-blowing too!

That is one of the amazing aspects of prostate play—a man can come without having his penis touched! This takes time and patience (familiar themes!) and an understanding of a fundamental aspect of male anal stimulation that can be worrying—the floppy.

When a man has something inside his rectum, he may lose his erection. While this can be disconcerting, it's not something to worry about. Sometimes this happens for the simple reason that their erotic energy is elsewhere. The sensations all move to the rear and the penis says, "Go to town back there, I'll come back on duty when you're ready." With some concurrent stimulation, you may inspire some fresh enthusiasm from his penis. If not, that's okay, too.

Some men find that they can have ejaculatory orgasms from prostate stimulation even when they're limp. This is a more advanced technique that takes a lot of practice to learn (for both the massager and the man), but if you do manage it, this kind of orgasm is both a physical thrill and a psychological wonder. Men are used to ejaculating only when they are hard. Accepting the new sensations of extreme stimulation without going to penile touch can be challenging. The catcher's hands might involuntarily move to his cock! (Which isn't necessarily a bad thing.) Harnessing these feelings and directing them toward learning to come without a hard-on requires focus, patience and training. Don't worry, though, the training is great fun.

Cocks—bio or dildo—are also great prostate stimulators. Depending on how your appendage of choice is shaped, the prostate can be tickled in either a missionary, doggie or on top position. If the receiver is on top, he can control the penetration and the motion against the prostate, which is a big plus, but it's great in any position.

Prostate massage is also very healthy. It reduces the risk of prostatitis and possibly prostate cancer.* It can also improve erectile performance and reduce the need for frequent nighttime urination. It's a winner all the way around.

Prostate play feels great and is also very healthy.

Now that the prostate has been revealed for the pervy pleasure point it is, it's time to learn about the unique and equally erogenous spot hiding away in women's asses. It's called the perineal sponge, and it's not a well-known piece of female sexual anatomy. A quarter-sized patch of erectile tissue, it's located in the wall between the vaginal canal and rectum and can be accessed from either orifice, about an inch or so inside.

Like all erectile tissue, the perineal sponge engorges with blood when stimulated. It loves attention when properly aroused. Rub as gently or firmly as your partner likes, from inside the vagina, ass or both! Try squeezing it with one finger in her ass and one in her vagina. This makes a great addition to oral sex.

Misconceptions About Anal Sex

While anal sex has increased in cultural popularity and prominence, it still carries some significant stigmas and challenges. Even though more and more people are discovering the wonderful sensations and increased intimacy offered by ass play, others continue to be victimized by misinformation and gender-role stereotypes.

The two most challenging misconceptions affect men and women differently and reflect socially constructed gender roles.

On the ladies' side, we're supposed to believe that women do not enjoy anal sex. Why? Because they've got a 'better' hole, a 'more appropriate' hole, in front.

This couldn't be further from the truth. There are women who don't enjoy anal just as there are women who don't enjoy swimming or sweet and sour soup. A lot of women don't enjoy bad anal sex or how butt sex is presented in porn. And there are lots of women who love anal play.

The fact is that women have excellent anatomical reasons to love anal play and penetration: There are lots of wonderful-feeling nerve endings in the anus, and women also have the perineal sponge to add to their delight.

*** At this point, the role of prostate massage in reducing the risk of developing prostate cancer is unclear. Not enough evidence has been gathered and cited to establish a true causal relationship. But it can't hurt to study on your own.**

Guy are getting the gender-expectation shaft as well. As men begin to explore their asses more—and it is becoming more accepted—there is still the nagging stigma that associates men and anal pleasure with being gay.

This is a huge obstacle for lots of guys. Straight men who might be accepting when it comes to other people's queerness don't want to think they might be queer themselves, not in the slightest, and when they have something up their butt and are liking it, this can get them wondering.

Guys, let's put it right out there in plain language. Anal pleasure is not what makes a man gay or bisexual.

Safer Anal Sex

The anus is tender territory. Its walls are not as robust and strong as a vagina and it is much more prone to small tears. Anal sex exposes both pitchers and catchers to the risk of sexually transmitted infections (STI's) and other infections.

Because we know that STI's can be spread from ass to penis and vice-versa, a condom is advised for anal sex. There is actually a term for not wearing a condom during sex (anal or vaginal)—barebacking. To bareback or not to bareback is something that should be discussed between the two participants because of the inherent risk. If you're in a respectful relationship, have been tested and have no apparent medical risks, barebacking is a reasonable option. You have to trust the other person completely, though. You're putting your health in their hands.

Condoms also serve another useful purpose in the context of penis-in-ass sex. With proper lubrication, condoms slide better than skin.

When it comes to other types of anal play, two other products are great for ensuring everyone's health. If you're thinking of fingering your partner's ass, slip on a latex or nitrile glove. If you don't habitually keep your fingernails neatly trimmed and filed, make a point of doing so before ass play. An errant sharp bit can do nasty things to a person's rectum. Ouch! Gloves provide a second level of protection against this.

Like condoms, gloves also have the added benefit of being slick and smooth. They can also be great to use while you're first getting comfortable with ass play or forever after as an easy hygienic way to play.

If you're into going down on ass, be sure to keep some dental dams on hand. These great, thin-but-sturdy barriers give you all the raunchy rimming sensations without the physical contact. Ass-to-mouth always carries a risk from STI and other infections. You can pick up dental dams at sex shops or order them online. Or you can use Saran Wrap, available at your local supermarket.

Finally, remember that all of these safer sex measures have yet another purpose—hygiene. Barrier products like condoms, gloves and dams can all minimize the potential of mess. Did you just pull a dildo or penis or finger out and it is a bit . . . brown? Just strip off that latex and problem solved!

Anything that goes in or near the ass must never go in or around the urethral and vaginal areas. Ever. This kind of sloppiness can cause vaginal and urinary infection, so either take a trip to the washroom for a soap and water scrub or do it the easy way and use barriers that can readily be removed.

The Cultural Shift to Anal

Anal sex is nothing new.

It might not seem that way, given the amount of attention paid to butt pleasure lately, but people have been seeking out those same butt delights for, well, ever. Straight, queer, men, women, people of every orientation and inclination have been having anal sex for as long as we've been walking upright (and probably before that, too!). And not just for reasons of pleasure: It's a 100% effective birth control strategy.

So why has anal been such a dirty little secret—and what changed?

For too long, anal was the sex that no one spoke of. It was rarely written about and even when porn started to get popular, it wasn't a headlining activity. Much of this collective hush can be attributed to the belief that it was only gay men who fucked ass. That stigma was enough to keep mouths shut (even if asses weren't).

But then something interesting happened. The porn industry got wise to ass! The people of porn figured out that its customer base didn't just want to see vaginal and oral sex. They believed people wanted ass . . . and they were right.

Anal didn't just become popular—it took off. It is now rare to find a porn film, be it indie, fetish or mainstream, that doesn't have at least one anal scene. There are even sub-genres: gaping, double penetration, ass-to-mouth, rimming and more.

This isn't entirely a good thing. It's helped anal to be accepted culturally, but it's also where people learn how to do anal and it models really bad technique. It's all about pound, pound, pound, the application of lube is rarely explicit, and all the warm-up time that's needed to get the ass ready for that intense pounding isn't shown (if it happens at all).

If you want to try hard pounding, gaping (spreading the asshole so that it's open) and extreme penetration, well then, go for it! But for the most part, we should not be taking our cues from porn. It's mostly for show, and extreme is what sells.

Yet we should also be thankful to the mavens of porn for opening the door to anal, as it were. It's become something people do and, more importantly, discuss openly.

The growing comfort with anal sex has helped break down the myths we discussed earlier—that only gay men have anal sex and women don't like it at all.

Because people have turned around, taken it and then talked about it, anal has become more legitimized and normalized. Not completely—there still is a mild aura of taboo. But the progress has been considerable.

We've learned that anal sex isn't something to be afraid of and that it can be a great addition to our sexual repertoire.

We're learning to do it safely, painlessly and ecstatically.

Does anal sex require some getting used to? Absolutely.

Is there an art to it? Definitely.

And the rewards? Priceless.

SEXY SUMMARY

Although attitudes are changing, negative biases toward anal sex continue to be widespread.

The two keys to great anal sex are lube and patience.

Pain does not have to come with the territory. It is usually completely avoidable.

Mess can happen, but it probably won't be a problem if you maintain a positive attitude, use gloves, practice good hygiene—and have an unstressed digestive system.

Prostate massage is healthy and feels great.

Women have erectile tissue (the perineal sponge) that can be accessed via the anal canal.

Guys, liking how something feels in your ass does not make you gay!

Slow is good. Slower is better!

NINA HARTLEY *is a pioneering feminist sex worker who is using her body in service to promoting a sexually sane and literate society.*

Active as a performer since 1982, her rock-solid commitment to the importance of sexual autonomy has fueled Ms. Hartley's career in adult entertainment. As a performer, director, writer, educator, public speaker, and feminist thinker for all, no matter their orientation, she's traveled the world to deliver her message. She believes that sexual freedom is a fundamental human right and welcomes the new social media opportunities for spreading her message of knowledge and empowerment to the widest number of people. She's the author of Nina Hartley's Guide to Total Sex *(Avery Press). Putting to use her B.S. degree in nursing, she and her husband, Ernest Greene have produced the million-selling sex-ed video series collectively known as "The Nina Hartley Guides" from Adam & Eve, currently in its 38th episode. Still active in front of the camera, she and her husband live in Los Angeles.*

ERNEST GREENE *has participated in the production of adult video for three decades as a performer, writer, director and producer. His body of work comprises over five hundred titles and includes some of the biggest selling X-rated feature titles in recent years.*

Greene is particularly well known for his groundbreaking approach to the presentation of unconventional sexuality related to consensual domination and submission. He has been active in the BDSM community for nearly thirty years, conducting workshops and seminars and serving as an officer of community groups.

He is the author of a new novel for Daedalus Publishing, Master of O, *which reinvents the BDSM classic* Story of O *set in modern Los Angeles and is told from the master's point of view. "Sexy, decadent, powerful and fun—exactly what you want in a date and in a book!" (Margaret Cho—Author,* I'm the One I Want*).*

CHAPTER FOUR

Power Exchange

by Nina Hartley and Ernest Greene

EDITOR'S NOTE: WITH THE STAGGERING SUCCESS OF *50 SHADES OF GREY*, power exchange (also known as power play, BDSM or kink) has crossed over from the wrong side of the tracks and become an approved game for respectable people to play.*

Historically, BDSM is associated with the infamous Marquis de Sade, whose name gave us the word 'sadist.' For many, kink connotes a brute in a basement with an unwilling woman and a whip.

This is not what power play is about. As practiced by knowledgeable people, it's profoundly consensual and egalitarian. And, because of its legacy, it's also territory that needs de-mystifying.

No people better equipped to do this than the husband-wife team of Ernest Greene and Nina Hartley. Ernest is a dominant by orientation who has spent decades developing his craft and teaching it to others. Nina, in addition to being perhaps the most famous porn actress ever (and a fine teacher in her own right), is an 'out' submissive, a direction inspired in no small measure by her relationship with Ernest, with whom she has been partnered since 2000.

Because there were two subject-matter experts in this chapter, I departed from this book's usual editorial style and set their thoughts down transcript-style. I felt this would serve them and the material better, and I also figured that readers would want to know who was saying what.

Defining Power Exchange

ERNEST: Power exchange is a form of sex play between consenting adults where, by negotiated agreement, one partner takes the dominant role and the other takes the submissive role. Once rules and roles have been agreed upon and the encounter begins, the dominant decides what will happen next and the submissive basically obeys.

*** The acronym BDSM stands for different things to different people. While there is general agreement that the 'B' stands for bondage and the 'M' for masochism, the 'D' can stand for domination or discipline and the 'S' can be shorthand for sadism or submission.**

Nina: Someone agrees to be Fred and someone agrees to be Ginger.

Ernest: The keyword here is not 'power.' It is 'exchange,' because all the parameters are negotiated in advance and nothing outside the agreed-upon parameters is permissible, while everything is permissible *within* those parameters.

Nina: This doesn't mean the submissive can't speak up if something isn't working or if there was some misunderstanding about the 'fine print.' If the submissive okayed flogging but neglected to mention that single-tail flogging is off limits, it's okay for that person to speak up during their session. They don't have to just wince and bear it.

Ernest: Refinement can occur during sessions, but the basic agreement is arrived at before the fun begins. The key point here is that, for all the talk about tops and bottoms—about power inequality—this is truly an egalitarian exchange. The partners meet as equals and agree on the rules of a game they'll be playing, Tops and Bottoms, the way kids in less politically correct days agreed to play Cowboys and Indians.

BDSM is done for mutual pleasure. The objective is for both the dominant and submissive to have an enjoyable sexual encounter that leaves both parties feeling happy, satisfied and tired in a good way when it's over.

Nina: That's not to say it can't be challenging emotionally or physically, or intense and profound, or personal and romantic. But the goal is still is for people to feel exhausted and happy at the end.

Ernest: Now, some people say that kink is about acting out power roles and that it doesn't need to involve sex at all. With all due respect, I think this is bullshit. This behavior is sex-driven.

Nina: Whether or not it's sexually expressed at that moment, BDSM comes out of a deep 'loinal' need to express something. It's fundamentally erotic.

Ernest: If you say that power exchange doesn't always end with conventional intercourse, that's a fair point. It's usually part of it, though. I'm pretty sure that in private, the overwhelming majority of people who engage in this behavior see it as an extended form of foreplay leading to conventional sexual acts that may or may not have some kinky accents. I suspect that those who say their BDSM is not sexual are either not telling the truth or engaging in some kind of strange do-it-yourself therapy.

A remarkable guy named Bob Flanagan was an important figure in the early years of BDSM's cultural emergence. He once said, referring to people who masochistically hang from hooks in quest of a spiritually transcendent experience, "If it gets too far away from what makes my dick hard, I'm suspicious."

I call this the Principle of Flanagan's Penis. If a given activity doesn't appear to have anything to do with sexual arousal, it's probably not BDSM.

Nina: Even if genital sex isn't the main motivation of people doing kink, and there are definitely people like that, the underlying motivation is still sexual. If a dominant has a submissive come in once a week to do their laundry and dishes, you can bet it's a turn-on for them both. The dominant's not just doing this because it's cheaper than maid service.

Power Exchange and Risk

Ernest: The physical dangers of power exchange are almost always overstated by people who have no experience of it.

It's true that some people do particularly risky things. They play with fire, knives, things like that—and they learn safe ways to do it. Just as there are safe ways to do movie stunts, there are safe ways to do edge play. If these people aren't very good at what they do, and very careful too, word will get out and they'll soon have no one to play with.

Most people do power exchange much more conservatively. Their notion of kink doesn't involve much mortification of the flesh. Typically there's a bit of bondage, a bit of spanking and then some sex. You still have to be careful, but it's not really all that risky.

On any given Saturday in a big city, a lot of people will be doing BDSM together. Yet if you stop by the emergency room of a local hospital, you'll probably find lots of people there with sports injuries, but no one with a BDSM-related injury. It's simply not that dangerous.

Whatever level you play at, you do have to be careful. For many years, the mantra of conscientious BDSM players was "safe, sane, and consensual." The phrase never quite worked for me, because how sane is it to wear latex in Florida in July? I'm more inclined toward a more recently developed acronym—RACK, for "Risk-Aware Consensual Kink." My point here is that with both these phrases, there's an emphasis on safety.

Nina: Ernest and I don't have a safe word because we don't do anything that's really dangerous. Still, it's important to stress the need to be risk-aware even if you're not doing edge play. If your partner has a bad shoulder, you don't want to restrain them in a way that'll make it worse. If your partner has bad knees, you might want to give them a pillow when they serve you.

Ernest: You never want discomfort to interfere with the 'torture.'

The Appeal of Power Exchange

Ernest: While Nina and I and many other people find kink compelling, it's not for everyone. We don't believe in proselytizing.

Nina: Like Ernest, I don't believe in talking anybody into anything. When I speak with people in the public, one of the most common questions I get is, "How can I get my partner to do such-and-such?" My answer is always this: Healthy sex does not involve getting anyone to do anything. It involves discussing things as equals and either reaching an agreement, or not. There's no place for chicanery, cajoling or 'talking into.' If you want to get your girlfriend to let you do her in the butt, you don't start there. You say, "I'm interested in exploring anal eroticism with you. Would you like to get a book and work on it together?"

Ernest: If you're interested.

Nina: Yes. If you're interested.

Ernest: One reason BDSM is popular is because it's caught a cultural wave. It's 'in,' it's hip and it's hot. Kink used to be relegated to a bad part of town that no sensible, self-respecting person would dream of visiting. Now the kink quarter is attracting lots of tourists.

Nina: The appeal can also be orientational. While power exchange is only one of many ways I can enjoy sex, Ernest's sexuality is entirely kink-oriented. He is a dominant heterosexual man who doesn't switch. For him, all sex has a power exchange format. He can dance any number of dances as long as he's the leader and she's following. He can dance the rumba, he can dance the cha-cha, he can dance the waltz. But he has to be leading.

Ernest: It's orientational for me at the same level as being gay. I have never had any real interest in sex absent power play. It's not that I'm totally disinterested, but it's like being a birdwatcher—it's mildly interesting but not arousing. If it were a question of 'normal' sex or no sex for the rest of my life, I'd probably read a lot of books and take up knitting.

For a long time, I was concerned that I was a freak, but there are actually a lot of people like me. The nature factory has a big kink wing. It turns out lots of us.

Nina: BDSM also gives people the opportunity to discover and express parts of themselves that might otherwise be repressed. Let's say I'm a feminist who believes that women are pathologically subjugated by our patriarchal culture. As a strong and independent woman, I also believe in pleasure on my own terms—and then I discover that what really turns me on is being on my knees before a dominant man. That'll give me some things to sort out, right? Kink gives people the opportunity to come to terms with who they really are, as opposed to who they think they should be. It's an honesty engine and, as such, it can help people become more self-loving and self-aware.

In my experience, BDSM is also a great container for creating intimacy. I have had sex with many, many, many men, and while I often had a fine time with them, Ernest is the only man I want to have sex with again and again and again.

Ernest: I feel the same way about you.

Nina: Why do I feel this way? Because something in me is being touched, and I'm willing to show it to him and he's willing to receive it and not stomp on it or make fun of it or whatever people do to each other when they're not being nice. I can hug and kiss anyone and lie on my back and they can have intercourse with me and I won't necessarily be touched by it. With BDSM, you can't do it well and not be there. You have to show up, and when both partners show up, you have the makings of something special.

Ernest: There's another possible reason for kink's appeal. In the evolutionary sense, we have two main urges. One is to feed and the other is to breed. Sometimes the two overlap—the female praying mantis bites off the head of her partner after they've had sex. BDSM may cross-wire these two impulses. If I tie up my submissive, I'm making it really easy to feed on her, the same way it's easy for a spider to feed on an insect that's caught in its web. Only then I don't feed on her literally. I feast on her sexually.

On the submissive side, if this hypothesis is true, there's something titillating about being prey. 'Eaten alive,' 'sucked dry'—in a sense, there's not a big difference.

Communication is the number one, two and three priority in power exchange.

Nina: Last but not least, BDSM can make us more conscious lovers. In a typical encounter, two people meet, are attracted to each other, fall into bed and have sex. Maybe they got drunk. Whatever the details, it just happens. They don't really talk about it.

A BDSM encounter can't unfold like that. It requires communication and negotiation. We need to know what we like, what we don't like and what our boundaries are, and then we need to share these things with our prospective partner. If I'm a dominant and you're a dominant, our bedroom tumble probably won't work out. We need to pre-establish that there's erotic overlap and discover where we're kink-compatible. All this requires us to be self-aware and to communicate actively. You can't just tumble into bed with anyone.

Doing Kink Well

Ernest: As Nina said, power exchange doesn't just happen. It unfolds inside a framework. Several frameworks, actually. The first of these involves negotiation and discussion. The partners need to communicate, and they need to do so before they go into their play space. In power exchange, this is the number one priority.

Nina: The numbers one, two and three priorities, actually.

Ernest: Yes. Power exchange requires consent, and consent means informed consent, and you can't have informed consent unless all the relevant information has been put out there.

Consent isn't merely the absence of 'no.' It has to be active as well as informed. Both the dominant and submissive need to step up to the plate as equals in a conversation that takes place before the action begins.

Some people believe it takes the heat out of things to talk about them first. And you certainly do want to leave room for spontaneity and improvisation. But that creativity needs to take place inside a framework where there are clear understandings about boundaries. If butt-spanking is allowed but anal penetration isn't, it's okay for me as the dominant to find out what the submissive's spanking edge is, but it's not okay for me to decide, since that butt is perched there looking so inviting, to just go ahead and stick a toy inside it.

Nina: These conversations need to go into detail. Let's say I want to experiment with breath play. That's okay so far as it goes, but what exactly do I mean? Maybe for me it means having your hand on my neck. We need to get clear on these details. Otherwise, you're going to put your hand over my mouth and pinch my nose, and although you believe you're playing within my boundaries, I'll have a full-blown panic attack and that's it, game over.

Ernest: With advanced practitioners, the conversation can be briefer. "Do you prefer thud or sting?" can cover a conversation about flogging. But they still need to have that conversation. If someone is unwilling to have a detailed prior conversation about preferences and boundaries, they are not a suitable partner.

Nina: In fact, when you go ahead and play with a person like that, that's when it can get dangerous. You need to choose partners who understand the rules and are willing to play by them.

Power exchange is enhanced by other structures, too. You need to create a safe space, a sanctuary, where you can play without feeling intruded upon by the clamor of everyday life. You need a space where you can show up and be fully present.

Ernest: Ritual and protocol are useful mechanisms for this.

Nina: Yes. They help you focus. For me, an effective way for me to get in the right mood for a session is to set up the physical space, prepare my body and get into my costume for the evening, which is usually pretty minimal but effective.

I look at it this way: Ritual itself is not sacred, but it allows the sacred to emerge.

Ernest: The container of ritual and protocol continues once the session has begun. If the submissive is required to wear a collar or always address their master as "Sir," or "Ma'am," these are protocols that establish the mood and reinforce the partners' roles.

While I'm a big fan of ritual and protocol, they can be overdone. When things get too fetishized, it can get in the way of intimacy and creativity. Power exchange is one-half about initiative and one-half about limits. The two need to be balanced.

Nina: Like a haiku poem or a sonnet, the limits create the space within which creativity can flourish. Once you build sturdy walls around the playground, you can play any game you want inside.

Ernest: Power exchange is a wonderful way to be sexually creative. Once you've got limits and a general sense of what the other person likes, then ideally there'll be some experimentation. You try this. And then that. And then this. There'll be some things you discover you both like. A session that holds no surprises for either person is, you know, meh.

Nina: You don't want to paint by numbers. Speaking as someone who likes being acted upon, what's fun about being in the submissive role once you're in the play space is giving up knowing what's going to happen next. Ernest puts it this way: The dom knows three steps ahead where they're going. The sub knows only the moment.

Ernest: Someone once said that the submissive hands over their nervous system to the dominant. That's a good characterization. The submissive surrenders to being done unto. That leaves the dominant with real power, which they need to wield wisely, and with an obligation to take good care.

Ultimately, the physical part of power exchange is there to reinforce an emotional gestalt. The biggest turn-on comes from inhabiting the state of being a top or a bottom. Everything else just feeds that.

Nina: This makes it important to stay in character. When you step out of character, you break the spell.

Ernest: If you make a mistake as a dom, well, that happens to everyone. Be nice to yourself when something like this happens—and don't step out of character to apologize. Just say, "Sorry, my mistake," and continue.

Some people are under the impression that being a dominant means you can't be nice or apologize or express emotions like affection. That's ridiculous. I wouldn't want to play with someone for whom I didn't feel affection. Dominance is a skill set I've acquired over many years with some considerable effort. I wouldn't want to lavish it on someone for whom I had no feelings.

Nina: It's not a contradiction for a dom to be loving. In power exchange, both the dominant and submissive are in service to their partner. When you strip everything else away, their basic contract is to delight each other. They're in service to each other and that's ultimately what makes the game fun. Since the top has already committed to being nice 'underneath,' why not be nice 'on top,' too?

Ernest: It's okay to be nice, but you don't want to be weak. Submissives don't necessarily want to be asked every other minute is they're okay or if what the dominant is doing is okay. The dominant's need for validation should not exceed the submissive's need for gratification.

Sometimes a submissive will make a sound like they're not enjoying themselves. You shouldn't ignore that signal if they seem genuinely distressed. But they may just be releasing into the physical sensation. You don't want to bring them out of their trance by saying, "Oh, was that too much?"

Nina: It's a delicate balance. When I was learning how to dom, I was often too solicitous. Ernest helped me learn to back off and not go every two seconds, "Are you okay? Are you okay?" Maybe it was my feminist over-training.

Ernest: To be a good dom, you can't be an inconsiderate jerk, but you can't be a wimp, either. You need to be okay with aggression and that's not easy. It took me years to accept this aspect of myself.

Nina: Ernest is completely comfortable with his bad self. He has no shame in his game. That allows me, in my submissive role, to really step up because I am stepping into a really great force field as opposed to something that's full of potholes.

Ernest: Aggression is an important part of what makes power exchange such a hot experience. A skilled dominant allows a titrated amount of aggression to come out and play.

Nina: It's not entirely up to the dominant, of course. As we've stressed, this is an exchange between equals—the submissive also has an important role to play.

Ernest: Being a submissive is an active role, just as being a dominant is an active role. If the sub has a problem with their shoulder and the dominant forgets about it, it's the submissive's duty to speak up and say, "Remember about my left arm." And it's the dominant's duty to say, "Sorry, I forgot about that. Let's do something else."

Nina: Remember what the contract is—to show each other a good time. To do that, the submissive has to participate actively.

Ernest: There is no honor in dominating a weak person.

Nina: Right—submit is a verb and doormat is a noun.

Ernest: In my opinion, the worst mistake submissives make is not communicating what they really enjoy.

Nina: The four words every dominant hates to hear are, "Everything's fine with me."

Ernest: Submissives get a lot of reinforcement for doing what they're told. Dominants generally get their reward in the form of the behaviors they exact, but they don't necessarily hear, "Gee, that was a great experience. I really loved it." A lot of people assume dominants don't need that, but that's not true. Like everybody else, they like to feel appreciated and to know they're doing their job well. A skilled submissive will actively communicate this both during the session and in aftercare, too.

There is no honor in dominating a weak person.

Nina: Doms need love, too.

Ernest: Yes, they do. I used to play with a submissive who could take very powerful stimulation. She would often communicate considerable suffering early on, well before she'd reached her actual limit. Eventually I asked her about this and she said, "I'm doing it for you. Isn't a response what you're after?" She was participating actively, letting me know that what I was doing was working. When I learned why she was doing what she was doing, I appreciated it.

It's not just the dominant who is playing with their partner's nervous system. The submissive is, too. Just as the dominant needs to know how the submissive is wired and what buttons to push, the submissive needs to know how the dominant is wired and what buttons to push.

Nina: There's a way for submissives to ask for what they want, or to communicate that something isn't working, in a way that stays in character and pushes the dominant's turn-on button instead of inducing what we call 'top drop'—the dom deflates like a balloon. It took me a while to learn how to do this.

Ernest: And you do it superbly.

Nina: What I've come to understand is that being a submissive is its own force field, just like being a dominant.

It keeps coming back to this: Power exchange is relational. You can only do what works for the both of you, and you have to take care of each other.

Ernest: Not everyone agrees about this. There are some absolutist dominants out there who go, "I'm the one in charge here. We're going to do it my way." I say, "No, it's relational." Some masters say, "I don't perform oral sex on my slave because it's just not appropriate." And I say to them, "Dude, you're making the sounds of a master who's about to be fired."

Nina: You want to be as fully present as possible when you do power exchange. This means paying very close attention to what the other person is experiencing. While this is especially true for dominants, it's true for submissives, too.

Ernest: This is why I don't like music during sessions. I don't want anything that interferes with my ability to attend to my partner's breathing, heartbeat and so on.

It's especially important to pay attention when you're working with your submissive's edge. Some dominants like to push limits. Some submissives like to be challenged. If that's part of your dynamic, fine. Personally, I prefer a more cooperative, collaborative model. I look to pick up subtle cues about what's working or not and how far I should go.

Nina: So if '10' is panic mode and 'five' is no problem, you might take it a bit past 'seven.' A little push is nice, but you don't want the person to start feeling panicky or out of control.

Ernest: An exchange might go like this. I say, "Are you interested in trying this?" "Yes, I'm interested in trying." We'll start at a low intensity and I'll build it from there. "How do you like this? How about this?" Eventually you get to a point where they go, "No, no, no," or they make some sort of noise or their body stiffens up. This indicates that you're probably at their edge, so you back it off a bit. Doing this requires you to pay exquisite attention.

NINA: The secret to being a good dominant is giving the right orders, and the secret to giving the right order is to find out what your partner wants to do. Then you 'order' them to do it. You give your submissive permission.

This is what's so great about my sessions with Ernest. He gives me permission to be transgressive. He gives me permission to want something that badly. He gives me permission to be in that much sensual overload.

Not only does he give me permission, he approves of it. He applauds it. The more I go into that transgressive sub space where I'm living totally inside my pleasure, the more positive feedback I get from him. It's a lovely feedback loop.

ERNEST: This won't happen if you play by someone else's rules. You have to be transgressive on your terms, in a way that's true for you. This is why it's so important to show up as who you really are. That's a big part of it, the willingness to say, "I've always been kind of embarrassed by my erotic attraction to pink tennis shoes. I've always thought it was kind of silly, but I happen to have a pair in my toy bag. Would you mind putting them on?"

NINA: If it's done well, BDSM creates an environment where you're witnessed and supported for being who you are.

Another thing I like about kink is that it can take you out of yourself. This desire runs very deep in our species—it's why we've been drinking alcohol and doing drugs for as long as we've been human. It's also why some people are thrill-seekers. If you go bungee-jumping or skydiving, you'll come out of the experience feeling you've gone through a portal, an encounter-with-death portal, and come out the other side. In power exchange, the submissive can go out of their head without getting drunk or doing drugs or facing a real risk. Core emotions around danger and abandonment are activated, but none of it is real—there's no actual danger and you're not going to be abandoned. You get to go through that portal in a context that's supportive and safe.

ERNEST: Nina and I like to say that power exchange is violence without anger, pain without fear and pleasure without shame.

SEXY SUMMARY

POWER EXCHANGE is an activity freely entered into and negotiated by equals.

EXCELLENT COMMUNICATION before, during and after the session is a must.

RITUAL AND PROTOCOL are useful containers that are ideally used to let creativity flourish rather than be constrained.

BOTH THE DOMINANT AND SUBMISSIVE have an active responsibility to do their best to please their partner.

POWER EXCHANGE is violence without anger, pain without fear and pleasure without shame.

JOSEPH KRAMER, Ph.D., *is an American somatic sexologist, erotic educator and filmmaker. In response to the AIDS epidemic, he became the foremost teacher of erotic bodywork in the world. He founded three important somatic sex education schools—The Body Electric School, the New School of Erotic Touch, and the Orgasmic Yoga Institute.*

Joseph has created 30 sex education films, many of which are available at his online schools: www.eroticmassage.com and www.orgasmicyoga.com. His most popular classes are Soft Cock Erotic Massage, The Best of Vulva Massage, The Joy of Thrusting, I Have What She's Having, *and* Your Junk is Someone's Treasure. *He was the first man ever to win the PorYes Feminist Film Award.*

For more than 30 years, Joseph has invited individuals committed to erotic liberation into communities of service. Joseph founded the somatic professions of Sexological Bodywork (www.sexologicalbodywork.com) and Sacred Intimacy, and developed worldwide trainings for these professions. Sexological Bodywork certification trainings are now available in California, Canada, Czech Republic, Australia, Switzerland, Spain, Germany and the U.K.

One of Joseph's current focuses is Porn Yoga for Porn Lovers. Porn yoga involves pleasurable, intimate and transformative practices that are done while mindfully masturbating to pornography. Joseph assists porn lovers in using their experience to enliven their body, open their heart, and create full-bodied orgasmic states.

CHAPTER FIVE

Touch

by Joseph Kramer & Carl Frankel

TOUCH: IT'S COMPLICATED.

And it's very simple, too.

As a trained massage therapist and someone who has been teaching massage and genital massage for decades, I know how technically complex touch can be. There are different types of touch such as tapping, stroking, pressing, squeezing, and caressing.

You can touch lightly or deeply; you can stay on the surface of the skin, go deep into the muscles, or work the areas in between. You can touch with your fingertips, your knuckles, the heel of your hand, your entire hand, your elbows or your hair. If you're being sexual, you can touch with your tongue, your genitals, all of your body. (Full body sexual touch is called frottage).

Touch can be calming or stimulating. Touch can be affectionate or even distancing. You can introduce yourself through touch and you can touch to learn about your partner. Touch can be used as a language. You can have conversations with others who know this somatic way of communicating. These are only some of the many touch possibilities.

So, yes, touch can be complex, but there's another level that's much simpler. I think of this level as residing 'above' the many technical options because it's about what's going on inside our heads. In many ways, the real action when we're touching is happening in our cranium.

The more focused and present we are when we touch, the better it will feel and the better it will communicate to the receiver. Inevitably, the receiver will feel how present we are, for better or worse.

Attention and Intention

After years of teaching both erotic and non-erotic touch, I've come to believe that the best way to learn touch starts with being mindful. Touch can be a powerful mindfulness practice. This means that we are consciously choosing to place our attention while we touch, and we are aware of why we touch. This 'why' is our intention as we touch.

Recent discoveries in neuroscience show that mindful practice over time produces beneficial changes in the middle prefrontal cortex. This part of our brain is associated with being empathic, controlling impulses, allowing us more access to insight and intuition, and many other benefits. I believe that my 10,000 hours of mindful touch as a massage therapist and as a Sexological Bodyworker have transformed my brain and me. I am especially grateful for my increased empathy. I call touching while aware of attention and touching while aware of intention the Great Medicine.

> *Intention transmits.*

We can compare attention and intention to a computer's operating system. Actions such as touch are like software; their nature and effectiveness are directly built upon and due to the characteristics of the underlying operating system. It's at the operating system level of attention and intention where we can learn to touch well most quickly.

As I've said, mindful touch involves attention and intention. When we direct and maintain our attention, there is power and sensitivity in our touch. Intention is the outcome we wish to achieve as a result of our attention. If we're touching someone, there are many possible intentions. We may want to give pleasure. We may want to arouse, which is a special, more intense form of pleasure. We might want to relieve the tension causing a muscle spasm. We may want to console someone with a hug when they're grieving.

Although we don't know the energetic or neurological mechanisms that make it happen, there's no question that intention is communicated through touch. Just think of all the individuals who've been offered a friendly massage and know from virtually the first touch that their masseur is really angling for post-massage sex rather than freely offering to give pleasure.

The Power of Presence

My focus on the mindfulness of both the toucher and the receiver reflects my belief in the transformative power of all forms of meditation, which are about learning to stay present regardless of what comes our way. The fact is that it's always difficult to be present. If it were simple, we wouldn't need to practice mindfulness. We'd 'just do it' à là Nike.

Intimacy can be threatening and touch is inherently intimate, so it can do an especially good job of sending us into our heads, even when the touch isn't sexual. Mindfulness meditations are a powerful way to become more skilled at staying present during touch. I often recommend vipassana meditation to individuals who easily get distracted during touch. In vipassana, you focus on your breath—in and out, in and out—and simply watch your thoughts go by. You don't judge them, and you don't get caught up in them. Thoughts are treated like items of clothing just out of the wash. You pick each one up as you notice it, hang it on the line, and then return to watching your breath, in and out and in and out. Vipassana meditation is one of the great learning modalities of our time. It makes us more skillful at being present, and great presence makes for great touch.

A friend in Switzerland has participated in or guided more than 100 ten-day vipassana retreats. A couple of years ago, he participated in a Sexological Bodywork training I led. He had never explored touch or erotic practice, but student after student in this training told me his touch skills were amazing. He was completely present with his attention and, because he was so present, he communicated his intention exquisitely. Every person he touched responded powerfully to him and it was due to the quality of his presence.

I have developed a multitude of somatic exercises that help people develop the ability to place their attention and maintain that placement of attention. One simple but powerful practice involves touching oneself anally. This is charged territory for many people because it feels 'dirty,' 'wrong' or 'forbidden' to them. I have my students lie on their sides with their pants or skirt off. The mindfulness practice involves oiling the groove between their buttocks, then slowly gliding the side of their hand back and forth in the groove for fifteen minutes. And staying present to the feelings.

Vipassana meditation is one of the great learning modalities of our time.

Fifteen minutes is a long time to be massaging the crack of your ass or any other place on your body. It can get boring and it can bring up distracting thoughts. The question is: Can you keep your attention on the sensations of hand caressing skin? After a while, most people's attention wanders because they're bored or anxious. This is why I recommend this exercise. It's an opportunity for individuals to practice bringing their attention back to the present moment, again and again.

In every physical encounter, whether it's sexual or non-sexual, uninspired moments happen. Boring moments can cause your mind to wander. Skilled touchers and lovers stay present during these non-peak moments. People treasure mindfulness, and they crave being deeply attended to. So presence is a talent that is highly appreciated. Not drifting away is not only a touch skill, it is a crucial sex skill—one you can learn through practice.

Technique Matters

I'm not suggesting technique is irrelevant. If your partner wants a vulva massage, specific skills are involved and it will help if you know them. There are universally applicable skills—how to enter a woman's vagina, for instance—and there is also person-specific expertise such as how this particular woman likes her labia to be caressed. There are many different ways to learn the first set of skills. You can take a workshop or find video guidance. You can extrapolate general touch principles from your partners' collective responses and feedback.

As for person-specific skills, that requires you to communicate with the person you're touching. You'll only know how Joanne likes her labia to be touched if she tells you. Or, better yet, shows you.

As a rule, showing is better than telling, and doing is better than merely seeing a technique demonstrated. I have two websites with over eighty hours of touch and erotic touch video instruction. Most of the demonstrations focus on technique. While I've come to believe that people don't learn much from watching, it can provide a good start. You see what someone else is doing and then you replicate it in your own practice sessions. Ultimately you learn by doing, with guidance from others who are skillful.

The Three Main Modes of Touching

Most touch falls into three categories. We touch to offer sensation, we touch to connect, and we touch when we are playing roles.

Each mode of touch calls forth a different type of attention. If you're touching to offer sensation, your focus will be on the point of intersection between flesh and flesh. You'll be noticing what feels physically good for your partner. If you're asking questions when you're touching for sensation—and I recommend this highly!—they'll be along the lines of "How does this feel?" And even better: "How could I improve it?" "Faster or slower?" or "More pressure or less pressure?" Since your partner is focusing on sensation, excessive speaking will become a distraction as soon as you find pleasurable touch. Repetition of these pleasurable strokes allows your partner to sink deep into feeling.

When you touch for connection, you often are not focusing on sensation at all. You are communicating with your touch. This is when touch becomes a language. You are paying attention to your partner's response to your touching and then you are responding with touch back to your partner. Your pursuit of connection might include visualizations such as sending love to your partner in every caress. Mindfulness is essential for connecting with a partner.

Last but not least, there's touch defined by role-playing. Sometimes we role-play like little kids at the beach, sometimes we role-play our fantasies, and sometimes we play professional or mythic roles. The term 'role' connotes many different things to people. As touchers, we are seducers, healers, massage therapists, lovers, consolers. We are speaking of authentic roles here, roles that allow us to go deep into touch.

I've played the role of massage therapist for thousands of hours with those who lay on my massage table. Both client and the massage therapist have clearly defined boundaries. For example, the client cannot initiate touch of the therapist. The therapist is allowed to touch this body part but not that one. My identity as masseur also defines my intention: I'm to touch therapeutically, so I don't seek inappropriate connections with my clients. The role determines how I touch.

Most individuals need to learn specific skills to play out the role of massage therapist. If they don't know the skills of that role, they can't offer all the possibilities of therapeutic touch. The analogy to Method acting is irresistible. You want to be the thing—you want to embody it, not just play at it.

There's considerable overlap among the intentions of touch, whether for sensation, connection or role enactment. If I'm touching my partner, I can be in the role of lover. This is fundamentally different than, say, touching them as a doctor would. I'll probably be aiming to connect as well. That's a role-play/connection overlap. If I'm massaging my partner, one of my main intentions may be to provide sensual or erotic pleasure. There'll be a role-play/sensation-play overlap.

As you go into a touch session, ask yourself questions about the role you're going to be stepping into with your partner. Will you be in the role of caregiver? Lover? Dominant? Submissive? Teacher? Student? Depending on the role, your mindset will differ. As your mindset changes, so will your intention and the quality of your touch. You may bring more authority to some roles. In others, your emphasis may be on being in beginner's mind and inquiry.

Two final thoughts about modes of touch. First, be sensitive to the possible consequences when you shift from one role to another. Let's say you're in the role of nurturer. You're holding your partner. You're stroking their hair and whispering safe, sweet sounds in their ear, the way you'd reassure a baby. You might not want to switch from there directly to erotic touch. It might land as a violation.

Second, it's a good idea to dialogue with your partner about what sort of touch you have in mind before you get started. If your partner wants sensation play and you want to connect, you're on a fast track toward disappointment and frustration unless you align your intentions beforehand.

Levels of the Game

As the toucher and receiver become absorbed into their experience, they become less conscious of the outside world. Touching for sensation, connection or playfulness can produce altered states in one or both of you. In our everyday reality, we experience ourselves as separate from other people. As the toucher, if you go deep enough into the touch experience, this boundary can dissolve. You find yourself in an altered reality, essentially a trance state. W.B. Yeats concluded his wonderful poem *Among School Children* with these lines:

O chestnut-tree, great-rooted blossomer,
Are you the leaf, the blossom or the bole?
O body swayed to music, O brightening glance,
How can we know the dancer from the dance?

When doing touch, you can arrive at a place where you no longer, as Yeats put it, "know the dancer from the dance." Boundaries dissolve. It's an altered state, a magical reality where you go out of your everyday mindset and into your fingers and touch. When you're in this consciousness, you don't have to think about what to do next. You know because your fingers know—and tell you. And the other person's body is speaking to you through your touch. This level of communication is available to almost everyone through regular practice.

You might expect inhabiting a role would make it more difficult, if not impossible, to enter this altered state. How can you lose yourself when you're focusing on inhabiting an identity? Well, roles create structure and order, much like the computer operating system mentioned earlier. They reduce our range of choices and provide a context within which to focus. If I know my role is that of massage therapist, it gives me a range of ways to touch and a range of ways not to touch. It simplifies things and this makes it easier for me to get immersed in the experience. Because I am playing a role, it's easier for me to go deep.

When you go deep, your kinesthetic (touch) intelligence is activated. Culturally, we have a limiting and inaccurate notion of what it means to be 'smart.' It's usually understood to be about cognitive processing power, about IQ. This is a school-learning model of intelligence and it overlooks the many other ways people can be smart. Educational scholar Howard Gardner has broken important new ground with his vastly more accurate and respectful model of multiple human intelligences. Among the types of smarts he identifies are social, logical, intrapersonal, musical, verbal and, yes, kinesthetic.

If you have a high touch intelligence, it's probably not news to you that your fingers can tell you how to touch. You already know how they can ask questions and get clear answers, too.

If you're not tuned into your kinesthetic intelligence, it may be because our cultural model of intelligence has gotten in the way. You didn't know more was possible and thus never developed your touch potential. It may also be that touch is one of your lesser aptitudes. The fact is that we're all stronger in some areas than others, and touch may not be your strong suit. If you don't feel great at touch, don't despair. Pretty much everyone can learn to go into touch trance. I know many people without a high kinesthetic intelligence who, with practice, became more adept than more naturally skilled people who didn't put in the time and effort.

The Fine Art of Paying Attention

It is the rare individual who is present all the time. Most us are present for a bit, then our mind wanders, and it either keeps wandering (from pillar to post to outpost and beyond) or we bring it home again. Distractions arise because they are something our hyperactive minds generate out of habit.

Here's what you can do when they come visiting:

- Notice the thought or feeling. This is probably the most difficult part—being self-aware enough to notice the distraction in the first place.
- Gently call your mind back to attention. Which, in this case, means being present to your intention and your touch.
- Be kind to yourself. Don't make things worse (and distract yourself more) by chiding yourself. Thoughts and other distractions are inevitable. Let them be.

Communication helps me to pay attention. When a partner guides or in any way comments on my touch, my attention becomes intensely focused. And my touch can help my partner to focus their attention. I have developed a series of mindful touch exercises that allow giver and receiver to communicate while going deeper into the experience.

Vaginal Mapping is my favorite mindfulness practice. This is not a massage. With consent, the giver enters the receiver's vagina and places one finger on the vaginal wall. The intention of the touch is to guide the woman's placement of attention to this one spot on the vaginal wall. The woman chooses the pressure and duration of the touch while reporting what she is experiencing. The giver might suggest deeper or faster breathing or ask about the pressure. When the woman is finished with the meditation on that point, she guides the toucher to a new spot on the vaginal wall. These mapping sessions often evoke deep emotions, memories, colors, and epiphanies. One finger held on the vaginal wall might bring up enormous resistance to going further. This mapping can bring to awareness a lack of feeling (called sensory-motor amnesia). In an hour of mapping, most women focus on ten or fewer places on the vaginal wall. If individuals without vaginas are interested in this mindfulness experience, I recommend Anal Mapping.

When it comes to touch, words can take you only so far. The real learning is in the doing. In these pages, I've laid out some directional arrows: 'Touch Mastery, This Way.' There's only one way to get there, though. You get there by practicing being present and by practicing touching. Touch requires embodied knowledge.

Our brains are amazingly plastic. No matter how old we are or how habitual our patterns have become, we can change and grow. We are the learning animal, and one thing we can learn—and keep learning—is how to become more present, how to become more compassionate, how to become more real. We can do all this by practicing touch while also reaping the immeasurably deep rewards of pleasure, connection and intimacy.

SEXY SUMMARY

THE MORE FOCUSED AND PRESENT we are when we touch, the better it will feel for both giver and receiver.

TOUCHING while aware of attention and touching while aware of intention are the 'Great Medicine.'

MOST TOUCH falls into one of three categories: sensation, connection and role-playing.

THE DEEPER YOU GO, the likelier it is that your kinesthetic intelligence will be activated and you'll go into 'touch trance.' This state is accessible to just about everyone.

TOUCH REQUIRES embodied knowledge. You develop touch mastery by practicing being present and by practicing touching.

Freeing Mind, Heart and Body

CAROLINE MUIR *has been instrumental in inspiring the modern Tantra movement in America. She is celebrated as a Tantra Yoga educator, best-selling author and transformational sexual healer for women and couples. Her Private Immersions are an opportunity to deepen the practices of Tantra in the privacy of working with a woman who has vast experience understanding the mysteries of the Feminine.*

She's the author of two best-selling books, Tantra Goddess, A Memoir of Sexual Awakening, *and* Tantra, The Art of Conscious Loving *(co-authored with Charles Muir). She's also the co-producer of the DVD* Secrets of Female Sexual Ecstasy.

Caroline founded the Divine Feminine Institute for Men and Women in 2004 and is now the solo educator and practitioner for Divine Feminine Awakening.

She teaches at Esalen Institute with Charles Muir each year and is sought after as a speaker and educator throughout the world.

For more information or to contact Caroline: Divine-Feminine.com.

CHAPTER SIX

Accessing the Lover Within

by Caroline Muir & Carl Frankel

BEING A 'SEX MASTER' IS, BASICALLY, THE SAME AS BEING A GREAT lover, so let's begin by examining what this concept, 'great lover,' has come to mean.

If you were to ask a random sample of people what they understand a 'great lover' to be, they'd probably say it means being good with your hands and mouth, having a hot body, or having strong recuperative powers if you're a man and being orgasmic if you're a woman.

What's love got to do with this?

Nothing!

These qualifications are strictly physical and technical. Here's an irony for you: In our culture, being a 'great lover' has nothing to do with love!

The language has it right and our culture has it wrong. The truth is as logical as it is neglected: To be a great lover, you need to be great at loving and being loved. No matter how technically adept you are, if you don't bring your whole self and an open heart into your sexual encounters, you're shortchanging yourself and your partner.

There's a wonderful scene in the movie Annie Hall in which the characters played by Diane Keaton and Woody Allen have sex:

Alvy Singer: Hey, is something wrong?

Annie Hall: No, why?

Alvy Singer: I don't know. It's like you're removed.

[A ghost of Annie rises from herself, and sits in a chair to watch]

Annie Hall: No, I'm fine.

Alvy Singer: Are you with me?

Annie Hall: Uh, huh.

Alvy Singer: I don't know. You seem sort of distant.

Annie Hall: Let's just do it, all right?

Alvy Singer: Is it my imagination, or are you just going through the motions?

Ghost of Annie Hall: Alvy, do you remember where I put my drawing pad? Because while you two are doing that, I think I'm going to do some drawing.
Alvy Singer: [gesturing to the ghost] You see, that's what I call removed.

The scene isn't famous only because it's hilarious. It's because it's so familiar. Lots of people have trouble staying present when they're having sex.

The meditation teacher Jack Kornfield cites a sign he once saw in a Las Vegas casino as a fundamental spiritual truth: "You have to be present to win." Indeed—and the same principle applies to the bedroom. You won't be a great lover—a sex master—if counter-productive stories and emotions block your ability to be erotically and emotionally intimate with your partner. The greatest heights of ecstasy are achieved when the physical sex is just one aspect of two souls meeting fully.

Let me be very clear about what I'm *not* saying. I'm not offering an opinion about whether sex without love is a good or bad idea. That depends on the circumstances and the partner. Nor am I suggesting that you have to be in a committed love relationship to have sex with another person. We carry the capacity to love inside us and can shine its light on whomever we choose. This could be someone we're married to or someone we met at a party earlier that evening.

But while I'm not judging, I *am* advocating. I want to bring the love back into lovemaking. When we 'make love,' we create something much more powerful than the pleasure that friction between bodies generates: We increase the amount of love that's in the world. We 'make love' in the same sense that we 'make a baby.'

So: If you want to be a sex master, you need to be a great lover. You need to be 'great with love,' another way of saying 'pregnant with love.' You need to be able to birth this love and share it with your partners.

In theory, it's a simple thing to open our hearts and love. In reality, it's not that easy. At some point, life hits us all upside the head with the lesson that loving is dangerous. As children, we love our parents and this relationship creates wounds that last a lifetime. Later, we fall head over heels in love with Mister or Ms. Right only to learn eventually that, oops, we erred. Our hearts go into lockdown or, at a minimum, get shielded.

The Garden of Eden is an archetypal place of perfect, unobstructed love. We all long to get back there, and we can. First, though, we have to clear out the internal blockages that keep us from loving as fully and freely as we might.

My life's work consists of helping people do this. For years, I taught Tantra with my former husband (and still dear friend) Charles Muir. One of the techniques we taught is sacred spot massage, a process that helps people clear emotional pain that's settled into their body tissue. My current work, while fully aligned with Tantra, focuses on the principle of the divine feminine. This archetypal energy inhabits all of us, regardless of gender. It's as powerful as male energy, but also very different. It's about surrendering, not possessing—you can't deliver a baby by holding onto it, you have to let go and open.

When men access their internal divine feminine, they become more interested in connecting and less interested in dominating. Not that dominating is necessarily a bad thing—there's a time and place for everything, including ravishing. But it's great to be able to enjoy the simple delight of being physically intimate with another person.

How do you access the lover within? By giving your mind a story makeover and by clearing emotional trauma from your body.

Shifting Our Stories

First things first: We need to let go of inhibiting stories we carry around inside our heads, such as the one I mentioned earlier, that tell us it's dangerous to love. There are actually multiple variations on this theme:

- The *love is a scarce resource* story. The notion here is that there is only so much love to go around, so we shouldn't squander it. It's as if we all have love bank accounts and the number's too low for us to feel safe, so we hold back on making withdrawals.

- The *love spins you out of control* story. You know how it is: You open your heart to a person, and the next thing you know you're head over heels in love with someone who may not be available, may not reciprocate, or may be a terrible choice. Love is like a bobsled run: Once you start sliding down it, there's no stopping. A million cautionary tales have been created from this narrative. Beware the unreliable heart!

- The *you should save your love for that one very special person* story. This wildly romantic notion tracks back to both the "love is a scarce resource" and "love spins you out of control" narratives. If love is a scarce resource, it stands to reason that we should save it—build up our bank account, as it were—for that one special person. And if love spins us out of control, then let it be with the one person in the world with whom it will be safe to slide down that bobsled run.

With each of these stories, we take a kernel of truth and then make the illogical (and very human) mistake of blowing it up into an erroneous general proposition that keeps us from opening our heart.

With the "love is a scarce resource" story, the grain of truth is that we didn't feel sufficiently loved as children—there really wasn't enough love to go around, or at least it felt that way. But then we transform "this is how I felt" into "this is how things are," and choose from that point forward to be ungenerous with our love.

The more rewarding view is that love is abundant. Mother Theresa put it this way: "I have found the paradox, that if you love until it hurts, there can be no more hurt, only more love."

Love truly is infinite, but we can't open our hearts to the reality of abundance until we open our minds to the possibility that it might be so. The mind leads, the heart follows.

The grain of truth in the "love spins you out of control" narrative is that when we open our heart, it's not only easier to feel love, it's also easier to fall in love, with sometimes undesirable results. The time can be wrong and the person can be wrong, too. But it's usually our 'stuff,' not love, that's the problem. Stuff like being unable to maintain healthy boundaries, or being obsessive, or hungering for validation from someone else when it's really ourselves we should be turning to.

The healthier and ultimately more useful view is that love needn't send us out of control. We all have the capacity to love without jeopardizing heart, health or hearth. We can admire, love and celebrate another person—we can even be in awe of them—without becoming unhealthily attached. Maintaining healthy boundaries is a learned skill, but it's achievable.

The "you should save your love for that one special person" narrative combines two stories—the 'there's a soul mate out there waiting for you' story, which has a lot of traction in both New Age and romantic-novel circles, and the increasingly discredited notion that you should be a virgin when you marry. The grain of truth here is that each of us is special. We all have our own unique beauty, and occasionally the veil drops enough for it to be seen.

We always have the option of looking for that special something in our partner, whether that person is our spouse or a casual encounter. We don't need to wait for that one person in a million to come along, and thank goodness for that. Many people are inspired by the idea of that one special person, but for me it's a scarcity narrative and sad story.

I totally resonate with the words of the priest and philosopher Pierre Teilhard de Chardin, who wrote, "Someday, after mastering the winds, the waves, the tides and gravity, we shall harness for God the energies of love, and then, for a second time in the history of the world, man will have discovered fire." If his words startle, it's because we don't usually think of love as a force of nature. But it is. It's one of the most powerful forces in the world.

Imagine a universe where love is abundant and it feels safe to love. That world exists—but we have to choose to step into it. That journey begins when we swap out our limiting stories for more generous ones.

OLD STORY	GRAIN OF TRUTH	NEW STORY
Love is a scarce resource.	As children, we experienced love as a scarce resource.	Love is abundant.
Love spins you out of control.	People without good boundaries can lose themselves when they fall in love.	You can love without spinning out of control.
You should save your love for that one special person.	Every person is special.	When you're being sexual with someone else, it's more than okay—it's desirable!—to look for, celebrate and delight in what's special about that person.

Healing Our Bodies

In addition to re-writing old scripts that don't serve us, we need to clear out the embodied memories and traumas that make us afraid to love. Like Annie Hall, many of us have troubling emotions that surface during sex. These feelings shut us down and isolate us. Our challenge then becomes to reduce the power of these fears so they intrude minimally or not at all on our connection with our partner and our pleasure. Over the years, I've helped thousands of people release their embodied fears so they're able to be more consistently loving and present while being sexual.

My own story provides a case in point. As a young woman, I was very curious about sex, but my experiences were less than satisfactory. The men I slept with didn't have the specialized knowledge that would help me open sexually. I then became interested in Tantra, which attracted me because it was about spiritual connection and intimacy. But then, as I explored Tantra, I discovered that there were parts of me that would shut down at a certain point during sex, short-circuiting my arousal and capacity to orgasm. Needless to say, this was very frustrating. For some strange reason, men frightened me—especially when they got lusty and powerful and erect. Their arousal made me uncomfortable.

I couldn't watch porn, either. The women gave blow jobs and this disgusted me.

I didn't want to keep having these negative emotions, so I began to accept the generous offers of friends in the Tantric community to do what's called Tantric (or sexual) healing. As I surrendered to this process, I began to remember the many uncomfortable moments I had growing up due to my father's unusual interest in me as a sexual female, even before I reached puberty.

It wasn't until my mid-forties that, with the help of psychotherapy, hypnotherapy and Tantric healing, I began to remember the violations I had experienced as a child. My father never put his penis in my vagina, but he did penetrate me orally, which explains why I was disgusted at the thought of having a man's penis anywhere near my mouth. I eventually came to realize that men frightened me because I was transferring my feelings about my father onto the men I shared my bed with.

Now, years later, my childhood history intrudes minimally on my sexual encounters. I've developed the capacity to keep my heart open and I am blissfully orgasmic. While the old fears occasionally surface, when that happens I take stock and breathe away the fear. This usually does the trick, and if it doesn't, I share what's going on with my partner so he'll be able to support me.*

My story isn't unusual. Research indicates that about one in five women and one in ten men have been sexually abused. And, of course, there are many other reasons for emotional withdrawal, too:

- Physical intimacy can trigger *emotional claustrophobia*—intimacy is experienced as suffocating and triggers the impulse to flee.

- It can trigger feelings of *inadequacy and anxiety*: "I'm not doing it right," "It's not getting hard," "My ass is too fat."

- It can trigger what might be called *fear of fantasy*—"My God, I just imagined slapping her breasts really hard. What's wrong with me?"

*** I highly recommend communicating with our lovers—in a clear adult way—what we know about our emotional landscape. It's easy to assume our lover intuitively knows everything, but that's never the case. If there are limits to our pleasure, our partner should be told about them.**

Physical intimacy is charged territory. We need to be able to deal skillfully with negative emotions when they arise.

And they do, in most of us.

The first requirement for dealing with difficult feelings is awareness. We need to acknowledge that these painful emotions are showing up and getting in the way. Confronting this reality isn't as easy as it sounds. When difficult feelings arise, it's natural to go into denial and pretend they're not there. We try to shove them back into the closet and hope our partner hasn't noticed. While this may in one sense succeed—women have been faking orgasms for millennia—in another it's guaranteed to fail because not owning what's happening is a form of deception and deception creates distance—always.

For me, anxiety in the bedroom showed up as a tightness in my belly and difficulty breathing. I had asthma as a baby and toddler when my dad's inappropriate energy terrified me. The butterflies started to churn and I would gasp for air. Everyone is different and has symptoms they can learn to recognize and honor.

We can find a place inside ourselves where it feels safe to love.

Once you acknowledge to yourself that this emotional noise is a problem, you have to decide to do something about it. This is a conscious choice, and it takes courage. Just as it's easy to go into denial when painful emotions arise, it's tempting to trivialize them as a freak occurrence that couldn't possibly happen again. You need to be distressed enough by your suffering to want to change. It's said that the truth will set you free. It's true here, but first you must find the strength to say, "This is my authentic experience and I don't want it to be a problem in the future."

And then there's the change process itself. As I said, psychotherapy and hypnotherapy helped me immensely. Conventional therapy was only part of my story, though. Hands-on healing made a huge difference. In fact, based on my own experience and the transformations I've witnessed over the course of decades with thousands of people, I've come to believe that hands-on work can accelerate the healing process and produce emotional releases that would take much longer to achieve, or not be achieved at all, with traditional therapy.

Healing occurs when energy is released that's gotten stuck and is getting in the way. This energy might be in the heart center—perhaps the person didn't do some needed grieving. It might be in the throat center because the person didn't scream when they were being violated or because they had to 'swallow' the fact that someone touched them inappropriately when they were a child. For now, though, let's focus on trauma that's lodged in the sex center, which is where it often manifests. And let's assume, as well, that it will be a hands-on healing.*

In both men and women, healing work focuses on the area known in Tantra as the sacred spot (also discussed in the chapter on Tantra). When it's massaged, it can lead to profound emotional releases as well as amazing physical experiences such as whole-body orgasms or explosions of light and color.

The sacred spot is accessed differently depending on the gender. In women it's found in the vagina, in the general area of the g-spot. Because of its energy, its location shifts. You can identify it by the spongy tissue and the ridges that almost feel like corduroy. The sacred spot will swell from beneath the surface. Often, a pulse can be felt by sensitive, slow moving finger(s).

In men, the sacred spot is in the anus. It's not the prostate—prostate massages are great, but they're not what I'm discussing here. The male sacred spot is much closer to the entry point than the prostate. Between the base of a man's testicles and his anus there's an area called the perineum. If you insert your finger in your anus and curl your finger down toward the perineum, you'll find a spot that feels kind of like a woman's yoni (Sanskrit for vagina). That's the sacred spot. Your partner will be massaging this delicate tissue—or, more realistically, pressing their delicate finger into it.

That's right, guys: Your sexual healing includes getting a finger up your ass.

All kidding aside, most men welcome an opportunity to relax in this region that is notoriously 'up-tight.' Women need to be very present with men while attempting penetration into this 'off-limits' region. Coaching men to breathe and make sound will help them relax and trust you. Assurances from you of your desire to enter them with your love also helps. Plenty of lube here is a must. Anal sphincter muscles are designed to say "keep out."

For many men, the prospect of anal penetration is a big turn-off. Not only is it often a new experience, but it can also trigger doubts about their sexual preference. If I like it, does that mean I'm gay? The answer is an unequivocal no. If having a finger in your ass feels good, it's because it feels good, end of story. The nerves in your anus don't care if you're straight or gay.

It can also be difficult for guys to accept a passive role and let themselves be 'done.' This isn't true for blow jobs, of course—in that context, most men are more than happy to lie back and receive—but sexual healing is different.

*** California is the only state in the U.S. that licenses people to do hands-on genital and anal massage. The people who do this are called sexological bodyworkers: They use techniques developed by Joseph Kramer, a contributor to this book. There are also unlicensed people who offer sexual healings. If you're intent on going down this path, shop very, very carefully. There are some great unlicensed sexual healers out there and there are also some dubious ones. If the healer you go to abuses your trust, it can re-traumatize you and increase your suffering.**

When a man receives an anal sexual healing, it's physically invasive, fraught with the potential for powerful emotional releases, and often accompanied by the conspicuous absence of that powerful symbol of virility, the erect penis. Being flaccid can be upsetting if the man's focus is on being manly, not on being vulnerable.

The rewards can be amazing, though, especially if you relax and let go. Over the years, countless men have come to me after sexual healing sessions and said, "What an experience! I've never known what it feels like to relax like that.

Typically it's a lover who assumes the role of healer.* This isn't the sort of thing you can easily do on your own. To move into the role of "healee," you need to go into your feminine, yin side and surrender to your sensations and emotions. It's difficult to do this if you're also being the active 'do-er.'

This isn't to suggest that you can't do healing work on your own. Among the things you can do are re-write negative scripts, explore your erotic frontier, and get comfortable with having a finger or toy in your anus. You can also give yourself a sacred-spot massage. But the more you can let go, the better, and it's much easier to do that if someone else is being the active partner. It's also validating to have a witness present for any emotional releases that may occur.

Healers, take care not to enter your partner's body prematurely. With women, there should be enough arousal for digital penetration to feel good. Use your middle and ring fingers together to lightly press or stroke her internal pole of pleasure (the clitoris is the woman's external pole of pleasure). Similarly if a man is on the receiving end: Use plenty of lube, take your time, linger at the entrance, and work your way in slowly once your partner's body has relaxed enough to make entry easy.

Take your time when you're massaging your partner's sacred spot, too. Pay close attention to the responses you're getting. In Tantra, we teach a variety of different sacred-spot massage strokes: I highly recommend learning these if you want to become highly skilled at doing sexual healing.

If a man is receiving the healing, feel free to play with his penis while you're massaging his sacred spot. He'll enjoy it, I assure you, and if he has an orgasm while his sacred spot is being massaged, it may be more than your standard male orgasm. Men can learn to magnetize their ejaculatory orgasm energy back to the finger that's doing the sacred-spot massage and from there send it up the spine and into the brain. That's when the real fireworks happen—full-body orgasms and visions of color and light. To make this happen, at the point of orgasm the man needs to breathe in and send that energy in and down to his sacred spot and from there up the spine instead of just letting it shoot out the tip of the penis.

There's no time limit to a sexual healing. You can take fifteen minutes or an hour or two—whatever works for you. Nor should there be any goals. Whether you're the giver or the receiver, don't aim for a specific outcome. Let the experience unfold and accept it for what it is. The receiver may have an overwhelming emotional, spiritual or sexual experience. It may also be quite uneventful. Whatever happens is what is supposed to be.

Remember, healers, that it's not just about your finger (or fingers). It's about all of you. Put loving energy into your touch and send it out through your heart. Always hold space for your partner: Support them to be fully present to what they're feeling, whether they're receiving in stillness or having a visibly mind-blowing experience.

People rarely emerge from a single sexual healing completely free of the past imprints that have accumulated throughout their lives. I've felt completely healed only to be surprised when the old issue surfaces again. This is pretty typical. The healing process is like peeling back the layers of an onion. You clear the energy and then you do it again. Eventually the charge diminishes until it stops being a problem. The spiritual teacher Ram Dass once said that he was still as troubled as ever, only now his neuroses were harmless little creatures instead of big scary beasts. Similarly with sexual trauma: It doesn't vanish, but it stops getting in the way. My own story provides a case in point: I've got the same trigger points I always had, but I've learned to manage them.

For those who view hands-on healing as a bit much, I should note that it's also possible to do sexual healing without the direct laying-on (or 'laying-in') of hands. You don't have to actually touch the sex center to heal it. You simply need to go near it. If the healer brings loving energy and intentions to the process, traumatic emotions can be released although the person being healed is clothed and there's only the gentlest contact or no touch at all. In our classes, we sometimes invite the man or woman who's receiving a healing to place their own hands over their clothed genitals. Then, with their permission, we place our hands over the person's hands that are covering their genitals. There are multiple layers of separation and it feels very safe. I've seen many releases happen through this process. Intention and energy alone can be enough to facilitate a healing or a release of something that no longer serves you.

Your chances of success are greater, though, if you do sacred-spot massage with the support of a loving partner.

Sexual healing has three main benefits. First, as we've seen, it clears out emotional deadwood, and this makes it easier to . . . well, to *not* be Annie Hall. The other benefits are perhaps a bit less obvious. When you partner with someone on a sexual healing, it's a very intimate experience—we can probably all agree that putting your finger into someone's vagina or anus is a lot more personal than going bowling with them. It's a bonding experience, all the more so if the active person holds space skillfully. Which brings us to the subject of trust. As a rule, women need to trust their partner to let go fully. If their partner earns their trust by being powerfully and appropriately present while she surrenders, this can have a big payoff in future sexual encounters because he will have demonstrated his *bona fides* as a man and lover. When a woman trusts her partner enough to surrender fully, that's when the fun really begins.

Embodied pain can be released through sexual healing.

For both partners.*

Last but not least, sexual healing is an exercise in letting go of what no longer serves you. It is an exercise in surrender. In our hyper-assertive culture, it's often difficult for people, especially men, to access their feminine side. There's nothing like a sexual healing session to help a person develop their yin aspect and learn to let go. This is a fine thing for many reasons, including this one: Energetic flexibility—the capacity to access both your masculine (yang) and feminine (yin) aspects—is a sought-after quality in a male lover.

* * *

If you take anything from this chapter, I hope it's these two points.

First, open your heart and bring your entire self to your sexual encounters. As Jack Kornfeld reminds us, you have to be present to win.

Second, do your best to get rid of the blocks that keep you from being fully present. This includes trading in your limiting stories for more abundant ones and clearing out intrusive negative emotions.

Doing these things can make you a great lover and true sex master.

SEXY SUMMARY

To be a wonderful lover, we need to love wonderfully.

There are two inner areas to work on—your mind (change your story) and your body (release held pain).

Sexual healing can help us release embodied pain and shame. So can other somatic modalities like massage.

The best sex happens when the heart is fully present and engaged.

* It goes without saying that the same basic principle applies to homosexual encounters.

KAREN B. K. CHAN *is all about sex and feelings. She is a Canadian sex educator, facilitator, speaker and emotional literacy trainer. BK/Karen is dedicated to sex ed that is honest, plainly spoken and emotionally relevant. Her background is in clinical sexual health promotion, and her foreground is in authentic communication, creativity, and healing.*

For the last 18 years, BK has worked with individuals, couples and groups in educational and counseling settings on everything from HIV/STI prevention and birth control options, to relationships and desire. She trains parents, teachers, service providers and other care professionals on sex positivity, diversity and justice, embodied learning and emotional intelligence.

Above all, BK believes in cultivating acceptance, empathy and courage, and always challenges her audience to become a little more of the person they want to be. She works at a municipal public health unit as a health promotion specialist, and operates her private practice, FluidExchange.org, in Toronto.

Her five-minute YouTube video "Jam" (which likens sexuality to musical jamming) has received over 70,000 hits and is used as a teaching resource internationally. BK's current projects include short videos (one about risk-taking, and others that challenge the idea of normal); emotional intelligence education in schools; a pop-up artistic video collaboration on sexual pleasure; and a children's book series on feelings.

You can find her and her work at Fluidexchange.org, and follow her on Twitter (@karenbkchan).

CHAPTER SEVEN

Sex as Improv and Creative Play

By Karen B.K. Chan & Carl Frankel

MANY PEOPLE BELIEVE THAT THE BEST WAY to spice up their sex life is by assembling a grab-bag of new tips and techniques from sources other than themselves. No: If you want your sex life to really kick out the stops, the genius comes from within. Learning tricks and skills without nurturing creativity can deliver short-term thrills, but it won't sustain you for long. Embracing your inner creativity is a deeper and ultimately more effective way to profoundly and erotically connect.

We are all creative by nature. Geniuses, in that sense. Just watch children play! They're endlessly imagining, trying, failing, feeling, sensing, laughing, crying. Making fun happen.

Children inhabit their creativity. Grown-ups, less so. It's not that people become dull, it's just that their creative pathways get blocked or overgrown. Gender expectations, the demands of maturity and responsibility, habits, perfectionism—these and other factors obscure the paths that connect us to our creativity.

One of my favorite workshops to teach is on how to have sex creatively, like the way musicians and performers jam together. People usually come to this class without knowing what they'll be getting. They're often bored with their sex life—things have gotten too routine. They want more stimulation, excitement, and fun. They believe that hot tips, new toys, best positions—technical guidance, basically—is how they'll get their desires met.

I don't give them what they want. Instead, I help them go inside and awaken their inner creativity. They come to the session looking to be given some fish. I give them a fishing rod and teach them to do their own fishing.

But what exactly is creativity? Ruth Zaporah, renowned choreographer and founder of Action Theater, an improvisational movement practice, puts it this way:

> *Another way to think about creativity is that it's not about being creative, but simply about being. 'Being creative' implies being other than who you are, when actually creativity is being more of who you are.*

Zaporah's improv movement practice does not have technical excellence as a goal, although that's a common outcome. It helps people learn to move as creatively as possible by integrating more and more of who they are into their movements. Action Theater teaches people how to be spontaneous in the moment—to follow the path of their authentic impulses. Where do you want to go? Where does this moment take you? If you ask yourself these questions often enough—and act on them, too—you'll start living more and more in discovery, and this will make you more able to jam, more able to be erotically creative.

And how do we connect with our inner creativity? A great source of guidance is theatrical improvisation, also known as improv, which is all about tapping into your inner spontaneity in a way that's both authentic and collaborative. While improv isn't usually understood as sexual, what I'm talking about here, basically, is improvising your sex life. Many of the following tips on how to activate your creativity are drawn from theatrical improv.

1. Practise "Yes, And"

The First Principle of improv is "Yes, and." It's shorthand for "Always be additive. Never undercut or negate." It's as important as it is because it directly affects the underlying energy of the improv. Contributions that negate in any way are inherently deflationary—they take the wind out of the players' sails.

In the sexual context, "Yes, and" helps to resolve the tension that arises when we experience our fantasies or desires as inappropriate. Guilt and self-judgement are huge turn-offs. It's erotically deflationary when one part of us says "Go" and another part says "Stop."

To be human is to experience nuance and contradiction, even (and especially!) when it comes to sex. I want to have sex and I want to go to sleep. I am attracted to you and I wish I wasn't. I feel shy about doing a strip tease and I want to get really good at it. By embracing "Yes, and," you give yourself permission to accept all your feelings about a given situation without experiencing pressure to be right, have things 'make sense,' obey the rules, or meet your own or others' expectations. Giving yourself "Yes, and" permission is a great first step toward flourishing erotically, especially since our deepest desires often have the charge they do because they're so taboo.

Our psyches are complex and often inconsistent. Creativity thrives in an environment that allows and makes room for our many contradictions. When we 'should' on ourselves for our private desires, it's an erotic downer and an exercise in sex-negativity.

I'm not suggesting you can or should act on all your fantasies. As Megan Andelloux points out in her chapter (*Role Play, Fantasy and Communication*), there aren't any mind crimes, but there is wrong behavior in the world. Honor your ethics alongside your self-acceptance.

INSTEAD OF: *I'm queer; it makes no sense that I love watching straight porn. I should just stop.*

THIS: *I'm queer and I love watching straight porn.*

INSTEAD OF: *I am unequivocally opposed to non-consensual sex. It is hurtful, wrong and unlawful. Yet I find it arousing to think about rape. This is so disturbing that I won't permit myself to have those fantasies.*

THIS: *I absolutely oppose non-consensual sex and I am aroused by depictions of rape. Sexuality is complicated, and I'm complicated, too!*

2. Stay Open-Ended and Process-Oriented

Another foundational principle of improv is that creativity is not goal-oriented. It's not about looking good or executing 'successfully.' When people excel at improv, it comes from their commitment to the process, from focusing on what they're doing and how they're being, not on where they want to get to. They succeed by attending to origin, not destination.

When we watch wedding-goers dance, we can tell who is working hard to be impressive, who is trying to not look foolish, who is dancing just to get it over with, and who is dancing for the love of it. Only the last ones are in the moment, in their creative flow.

In sex, open-endedness means not gunning for orgasms (yours or another person's). It also means not being staunchly inflexible about your notions of what should happen next. Planning is great as long as it increases the possibilities and doesn't limit them. So bring those feathers to the scene! Just don't be stubborn about what time feather play happens or making it happen no matter what.

When it comes to creativity, curiosity is a better friend than achievement. Keep wondering what you might do, how something might feel, what might happen, how a partner might react. If you catch yourself thinking, "This better blow his mind, everyone loves this," replace it with, "Many people love this—what about him?"

The best goal is no goal. Being open to possibility is an exercise in mindfulness. During one of my brief but life-changing forays into meditation, I learned this important lesson: The point of waiting is to . . . wait. 'Success' comes from being present to the experience of waiting, not from the arrival of the bus, or sleep, or orgasm. Thus the point of a caress is to touch, the point of getting naked is to be naked, the point of licking the perineum is to touch it with your tongue. Everything that happens after that (arousal? sex? conversation? orgasms? laughter?) is a 'success' and part of your creative play.

The best goal is no goal.

The next time you're playing sexually, I invite you to check in with yourself about how open-ended you're being. Notice if you feel disappointed or resentful about how a certain experience turns out. It's a clue that you could become more process-oriented.

INSTEAD OF: *Once we've gotten naked, I'm going to sit on top, then I'm going to lean over and lay that big sexy move on him. Oh shoot, he's not sitting down! What do I do now?*

THIS: *Now I'm naked. Now I'm on top. Now I'm leaning over. Oh, he's trying to stand up, is he? Well, I'm going to cover his eyes!*

INSTEAD OF: *I hope she thinks I'm really good at this and tells all her friends.*

THIS: *Does she like this? Let me find out what part she likes the most.*

INSTEAD OF: *Where's my orgasm? I'd better orgasm soon. Am I broken?*

THIS: *What am I feeling in my body? In my bones? Do I feel an orgasm rising?*

3. Be Okay with Imperfection

You can't insist that a sexual experience be great. But you can create a space where it's easy for greatness to rush in.

Sex is messy, awkward and full of surprises. Unlike movies and porn, real-life sex is unedited and involves adjusting limbs gone numb, asking for whispered words to be repeated, fumbling with condoms or toys, bathroom and water breaks, exiling the dog/cat/ferret, sharing bodies from their most and least flattering angles, and so on. And, oh, did I mention farting? To expect your sex to feel, look, sound, smell, taste, or otherwise be perfect is to set yourself up to fail.

Real-life sex is imperfect. You'll have more fun—a lot more fun!—if you get comfortable with this. Let imperfection be your norm. Here too, don't 'should' on yourself. By cultivating an imperfection-friendly attitude, you actually increase the likelihood that those wondrous, perfect-feeling, star-aligned moments will occur.

Contrary to common belief, perfectionism is less about the pursuit of excellence than it is an attempt to control what feels out of our control. It's a way to keep from feeling bad, unworthy or ashamed. Where there is perfectionism, there is often also shame—it's perfectionism's flip side.

The best way to deal with shame is with patience, kindness, and compassion.. And so, when you bump up against your own perfectionism—when you worry about being not good or sexy enough, not experienced or confident enough, not masculine or feminine enough—take a breath and keep going. Offer yourself the love and acceptance you might give someone you love.

We are all imperfect—perfectly imperfect.

INSTEAD OF: *I expect the sex I have to look like it does in movies.*

THIS: *I expect sex might be messy, awkward, and full of surprises—and I delight in it!*

INSTEAD OF: *I carefully calibrate the sounds I make during sex. I don't want to come off too tame or too crazy, too loud or too timid, too high-pitched or too much like a beast.*

THIS: *The noises I make during sex are not pre-meditated. I don't judge how my vocalizations sound.*

INSTEAD OF: *I don't want to have to say what I want. Why can't my partner just know? Talking about it ruins it.*

THIS: *No one's a mind-reader. I'm am happy to tell my partner what I know of I want. We'll keep on trying to understand each other.*

4. Be in First-Person

Imagine watching someone dance at the wedding mentioned earlier. Imagine her being preoccupied by how his dancing looks to the photographer and the other wedding-goers. Then imagine him gradually getting into the groove, becoming less preoccupied until he loses himself in the trance of dancing. What you've just witnessed is the dancer transitioning into the first person. His inner monologue went from being inside the photographer's head ("Look at him dance") to being inside his own experience ("This feels amazing").

We call this 'losing ourselves,' but it's really more about finding ourselves.

Many people struggle to stay in first person during sex. They see themselves as if through a camera in the room. To varying degrees, they're aware of what they look, smell, taste, sound, and feel like to others. This is especially common for people socialized as girls and for survivors of sexual violence. For obvious reasons, watching a lot of porn can also coax your reference point outside your body—the watching perspective becomes ingrained.

I call this experience "third-person sex." It's characterized by a prioritized identification with who's looking at us along with hyper-vigilance about how others are experiencing us. Many people have third-person sex some or all the time. Some switch their reference points back and forth, others have third-person sex only with certain partners, some did when they were young but no longer—and some stay in the sexual third-person for their entire lives.

There's nothing inherently wrong with third-person sex. It can be a truly pleasurable experience. It's also possible to be a fabulous lover from the third-person vantage point—you're focusing on your partner's experience, after all, and this is one of the keys to being a great lover.

Third-person sex only becomes a problem when it starts getting in the way of your own pleasure. If you don't feel true to yourself or satisfied with what you're experiencing, or if you can't shift to a first-person perspective when you'd like to, then it's something to take a closer look at.

Third-person sex can also be a problem for partners. Common complaints might sound like "We go through the motions, but you're not really there" and "I just don't feel like we're connecting."

First-person sex is very much about being present, an intangible concept that defies definition—although, as with the famous definition of pornography, you know it when you see it (or feel it). If third-person is your habitual state, the perspective likely feels totally normal, and you may not even know that there may be something to work with here. Like they say, the fish isn't aware of the water they swim in. To shift into first person, the first thing you need to do is recognize that this alternative exists. At that point, moving your gaze from the corner of the room (or from behind your lover's eyes) to behind your own eyes will require some practice—and, quite possibly, some unlearning. You're learning a new habit, a habit of perspective.

Being fully present means being fully in the present, not in the past or the future. It means not planning or worrying (future), and not reliving a memory (past) as if it were happening now. Being present means tuning into your feelings and sensations at least as much as your thoughts. It means not getting caught up in interpretations of what you're experiencing. We are the meaning-making animal—we can't help but create stories that make sense of our experience. We can know a story for it is, though—one interpretation among many. Ground yourself in the sensory experiences that bring the story.

If, during sex, you find yourself in third person when you want to be first person, try shifting your perspective by practicing bodily awareness. Notice what your body is doing and what it's experiencing. How are you breathing? What is its pace, depth, sound? Is it cool or warm? If your body is touching another body, what does that feel like? (Not how should it be feeling, or what do you expect it to feel like, but what do you actually feel?) Tune into the quality of any motions you or your partner makes.

Be present to your environment, too. What's the quality of the light? What smells can you detect? As much as possible, notice what you're sensing without overlaying any meanings or stories onto them. "The air is cold" is a first-person noticing of your sensory experience. "I should have closed the window" is a story that takes you away from your direct experience.

Keep finding your way into your body. Your senses will take you there.

INSTEAD OF: *How does my butt look? If I stay upright, my partner won't see it in all its hideous glory.*

THIS: *I can feel goose bumps on my butt, the hairs are so sensitive!*

INSTEAD OF: *During sex, I have a complete picture of what's going on in the room at all times.*

THIS: *During sex, along with my thoughts and fantasies, I spend a lot of time in the first person, experiencing sensation.*

5. Get Comfortable with Discomfort

When you are present in first-person, you will not know how you appear at all times because you'll be inside looking out, not outside looking in. You'll need to trust that you are acceptable and desirable exactly as you are, without trying. This is something that many of us—most of us—struggle with. Awkwardness, self-doubt and self-consciousness are markers that you're human, not inferior or broken. They aren't problems unless they keep you from venturing into uncertainty, from allowing yourself to experience novelty.

Unless they keep you from growing.

A great way to overcome self-doubt and build self-confidence is by taking small risks. Trust in yourself doesn't come from burrowing down into your cave—it comes from taking small chances and coming out feeling intact and courageous.

The problem with risk-taking, of course, is that it's risky. You can't be sure how things will turn out—you're going into a zone where there will be uncertainty at a minimum, quite possibly discomfort, and maybe outright anxiety or fear. To proceed, you have to be okay with these feelings. Even better, you can befriend them as helpful emotions, as companions you ride with when you're being courageous. With practice, emotions that are hard to bear become more bearable.

You don't want to overdo your risk-taking, of course. If you're going to be jumping out of an airplane, you want to be wearing a parachute, right? With sex, too, you don't want to set yourself up to fail. You want to take risks that are calibrated to help you grow without having you end up feeling irreparably hurt or humiliated.

When I teach this subject, I find it useful to divide our experiences into three categories—the Comfort, Stretch and Panic zones.*

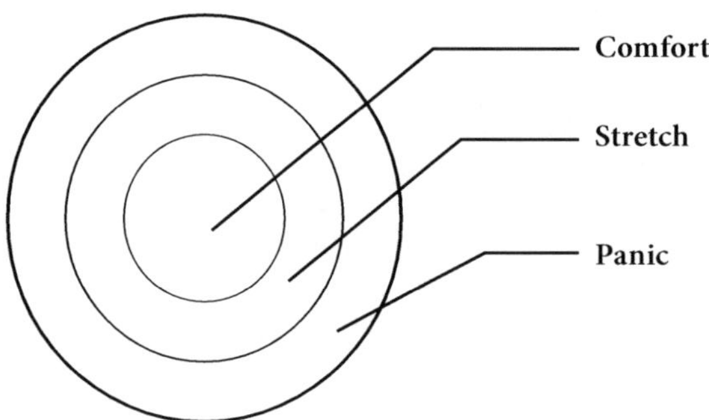

The Comfort zone, tucked in the core, encompasses all that is easy, habitual, known, and free of risk. This might mean kissing someone you know well, having sex that doesn't strain your back, talking and caressing after sex, or having solo sex. (And then again, it might not—what feels comfortable differs for every person.) Your Comfort Zone probably shifts from moment to moment and mood to mood. It may expand when you're well-slept or with a trusted partner, and shrink when you're feeling sick or unattractive.

Both the other zones—Stretch and Panic—involve discomfort. The difference between them is in your capacity to take in information, respond, and adapt. In the Panic Zone, the outermost circle, you're in fear-driven fight/flight/freeze

---

*** I learned of this model from YES!, an organization that promotes conscious social change projects around the world.**

mode. You feel highly stressed and shut down, and unable to take in information. You may feel ashamed, hurt, disgusted, angry or numb. Sexually, you may feel the urge to stop everything or to go into autopilot to "get it over with."

With courage, calm, and awareness, the Stretch Zone can be experienced positively, unlike the Panic Zone, where the adrenaline is overflowing and it simply isn't fun. In the Stretch Zone, you feel challenged, maybe by a new situation or partner. You may feel self-conscious, unsure or shy, but you are still engaged and present. You're listening, observing, and responding.

The Stretch Zone is the only place where we learn and grow—it has the name it does because time spent there will expand your Comfort Zone. Lifelong learners spend a lot of time in the Stretch zone—it's where a person's creativity is most active and alive. Sex masters spend a lot of time there, too.

When you're in the Panic Zone, you can't be creative, nor can you change that it is your Panic Zone. Growth doesn't happen here. Instead, take small steps into the Stretch Zone from the Comfort Zone. Ease off, and repeat. If the thought of being seen naked while having sex sends you into the Panic Zone, you might try being seen naked briefly, or partly naked—or you might try getting naked with people you're not being sexual with.

It can be very rewarding to take a trusted companion with you on these healing explorations. A great sexual partner is a friend, cheerleader, guide, and witness to their lover's Stretch Zone experiences. If you don't like your belly to be touched or even mentioned because you fear it's unattractive, you can begin to stretch that boundary by placing a trusted partner's still hand on it, and removing that hand after a while. The goal is to dip a toe into the scary places while staying in your Stretch Zone.

Like I said: Small steps, repeated.

In our lifelong journey towards authentic and creative sexual expression, healing can be both a motivator and a happy by-product. It allows us to live in more and more parts of the house that is our psychic home.

Instead of: *I don't do anything that might make me feel self-conscious.*

This: *When I trust my partner and am curious about something, I try it even if it makes me feel self-conscious.*

Instead of: *I'm not comfortable with talking dirty. I never have been and I never will be. It's stupid.*

This: *I feel nervous and judgmental thinking about talking dirty. What do you mean by 'talking dirty?' What are the different ways people do this?*

6. Fall Into the Gap

Life is a never-ending dance between routine and novelty. We are engaging our creative self when we take note of what's customary. By noticing what is usually invisible or taken for granted, we are already creating novelty.

Dancers discuss this dynamic in terms of what they call 'the gap.' Let's say a dancer routinely spins to the right when their arms are in the air. They open a door to new possibilities when they spin to the left instead. The turn may feel unpractised or awkward, or it may flow smoothly. The arms may stay lifted or they may not. The point is, everything they do from that point on changes, even in the smallest ways. When they do that, they're falling into the gap.

Stay curious and in learning mode.

Learning how to fall into the gap starts with noticing what our automatic habits are. We have lots of them. You unbuckle the seat belt as you turn off the engine. You tilt your head up and close your eyes before a kiss. You grasp the breast, then hone in on the nipple. The gap opens when we notice what we're doing. It opens even wider when we consciously choose to do something different. It might mean waiting till the engine's off before unbuckling your seat belt. It might mean keeping your eyes open when you kiss. It might mean caressing the breast without touching the nipple at all.

The same principle holds true with regard to your path to orgasm. We tend to know what works for us and to follow that path. Cheese at the end of the tunnel—good! There's a downside to this, though. That path can become a rut. You can learn new pathways to orgasm—we all can!—but to do that, you need to step off the known path.

You have to fall into the gap.

INSTEAD OF: *We usually have sex the same way. I climb on top and start moving. Then we turn over and I work my way towards orgasm on my back.*

THIS: *We usually have sex the same way. Today I'm going to climb on top and then not move. Instead I'm going to touch myself and see what happens!*

7. Enhance Your Erotic Vocabulary

While great technical skills do not a great lover make, great lovers usually have great technical skill. Being authentically creative doesn't mean you shouldn't pick up new toys, knowledge or skills. It means you can incorporate them playfully without relying solely on them for fulfillment.

When beginners think they've run out of moves, often what they've run out of is curiosity. One thing that differentiates the expert improviser is that they can stay 'in the investigation' much longer than a novice—they're adept at being curious and present. Even moments of stillness or repetition are rich with creative opportunity, especially if we can quiet those inner voices that criticize, fret, or complain about things getting boring..

I encourage you to stay curious and in learning mode. Read about the vulva's inner erectile network. Do Stretch Zone work on giving great head. Acquire new toys—or invent them! Masturbate while dangling off the bed and having all the blood rush to your head. Take bits from the porn that turns you on and try them (in person or in your imagination). Bring your curiosity to your lovers—make them your teachers as well as your fellow students. Learn about sex and sexuality from how people talk about their desires. Watch how animals court—what works for them may work for you! All this is grist for your mill and helps you expand your erotic vocabulary. New moves are a fine thing. They are not the answer, but they help us keep asking questions.

INSTEAD OF: *I know enough about sexual desire and pleasure.*

THIS: *When it comes to sexual desire and pleasure, I am always learning and unlearning.*

* * *

Carving and tending your creativity pathways is a lifelong form of play and practice. It is never too late to begin or to pick up where you left off. All that you'll need for the journey is already within you. And the fun is all in the travelling!

SEXY SUMMARY

PRACTICE "Yes, and."

STAY OPEN-ENDED and process-oriented.

BE OKAY with imperfection.

BE IN FIRST-PERSON.

GET COMFORTABLE with discomfort.

FALL INTO THE GAP.

ENHANCE your erotic vocabulary.

CHARLIE GLICKMAN, PH.D. *is a sex and relationship coach, writer, blogger, teacher and internationally-acclaimed speaker. For over twenty years, he has spoken at academic conferences and community events, taught workshops about sexuality, pleasure, sexual practices and relationships, and worked with individuals, couples and groups to help them have great sex. In addition to his work with the public, Charlie trains sexuality educators, medical and mental health professionals, and clergy to enable them to better serve their clients and communities.*

Charlie's areas of focus include sex and shame, sex-positivity, queer issues, masculinity and gender, communities of erotic affiliation, and many sexual and relationship practices. He is one of the co-authors of The Ultimate Guide to Prostate Pleasure: Erotic Exploration for Men and Their Partners, *the first book that explains the amazing pleasures of the prostate (also known as the male G-spot) and all the ways that men and their partners can explore its erotic potential.*

As a sex and relationship coach, Charlie works with people in person and over Skype to help them move past whatever is blocking them and make sex more pleasurable. He also coaches sexuality professionals who want to expand their skills and grow their businesses. You can find out about his services at MakeSexEasy.com, read his work at CharlieGlickman.com, or follow him on Facebook and Twitter as CharlieGlickman.

CHAPTER EIGHT

Sex and Shame

by Charlie Glickman & Carl Frankel

No matter how skilled you are, things won't always go as you'd hoped in the bedroom. A move that usually works wonderfully falls flat. You put your hand on her genitals and she moves it away. You spend way too much time worrying about how your ass looks. You ejaculate too soon. Your equipment won't operate as it's meant to.

We all hit these speed bumps sometimes, sex masters included. When it happens, a frequent response is shame—a sense of unworthiness accompanied by feelings of isolation and disconnection.

Because being ashamed feels, that's right, shameful, we tend not to acknowledge or discuss it. It's the great unmentionable, the red-faced elephant in the bedroom.

Our reluctance to surface shame is cultural as well as personal. If you have a rage problem, it's easy to find anger management counseling. If you're mourning the loss of a loved one, you can find a grief counselor nearby. But where oh where is the shame counseling? True, this is what therapists spend much of their time doing, but it hasn't been codified into a shorthand phrase. As a society, we're not yet honest or adult enough yet to give shame the attention it deserves.

Although shame is inevitable, it needn't be an obstacle. If we manage shameful feelings skillfully when they arise, we quickly regain our sense of connection and the erotic dance continues with hardly a misstep. But if we're not adept at managing our shame, it's all too easy to get lost in our pain and that's the end of fun in bed.

Figure skating is a glorious blend of artistry and athleticism. Even Olympic champions fall sometimes, though. Stumbles and pratfalls are part of the game. Do these highly skilled specialists train for events assuming nothing can possibly go wrong? Or do they and their coaches prepare for the inevitable mishaps? We all know the answer to that one. World-class figure skaters don't only practice axels and toe loops—they also become skilled at managing their emotions when things go wrong. They learn to regain their poise and focus as quickly as possible. They develop what I call shame resilience.

Not everyone can be Katarina Witt or Evgeni Plushenko, but we can all learn to be shame-resilient during lovemaking. That's what this chapter is about—how to skillfully manage feelings of embarrassment or distress when they arise in the bedroom.

Fifty Shades of Shame

Shame is the feeling we get when we believe we've fallen short of an expected standard of behavior. I'm at a fancy dinner party and I use the wrong fork for the salad. Someone points out my faux pas and I feel embarrassed. I should have known which fork to use—and I didn't. My bad, my shame.

There is a fair amount of professional disagreement about the meaning and parameters of shame. Here's a brief summary of my views.

An Inclusive Term. As I use the word shame, it includes an entire gamut of emotions ranging from mild chagrin to "I don't deserve to be alive" feelings of personal humiliation. Other experts define shame more narrowly. For them, it's a point on a continuum, not the entire continuum—embarrassment, for instance, is a milder emotion than shame. I find an inclusive definition more useful because it shows the commonalities across the spectrum of the emotion. Mild worry, fear, anxiety, and panic are on a continuum and share similar traits. Ditto for chagrin, guilt, humiliation, and shame. When we can see the similarities among these emotions, it becomes easier to develop inclusive strategies for dealing with them.

Not a 'Bad' Emotion. Some people use "shame" to refer specifically to the toxic form of the emotion—the one that says "I am a bad person," as contrasted with guilt ("I did a bad thing"). The notion here is that while guilt can motivate positive change, shame shuts us down. While I agree that this can be a useful distinction, I don't use the terms this way because when we demonize one of our emotions, we demonize a part of our selves, and ultimately we want to love and heal, not hate, ourselves.

Levels of Shame. Shame can be narrow and event-specific or it can cut broader and deeper. If my partner has prepared a wonderful Valentine's Day dinner and I space out about our date, I will probably feel bad about my oversight and ashamed that I forgot. But it won't carry any deeper messages about my fundamental worthiness unless I do this sort of thing often and have a story in my head about its making me a bad person.

Now let's take another example. Let's say I grow up with strong homosexual urges among people who believe that homosexuality is unnatural and perverted. The chances are pretty good that I'll grow up feeling abnormal and ashamed of who I am. Here, the shame goes deep. It cuts to the core of who I am. If I'm going to come out successfully, I'll need to exorcise my sense of unworthiness from a place deep in my soul.

A Social Emotion. We all internalize cultural standards about who we should be, how we should behave and what constitutes competence and excellence. Shame arises when we fail to meet those standards, when we believe we've fallen short in the eyes of people who share these norms.

This doesn't mean someone else has to be present for us to feel shame. We all internalize cultural norms (sometimes as a first step to rejecting them). If I believe it's unworthy to masturbate, I may feel shame when I spend an hour doing it although no one knows I'm doing it but me.

We can also feel shamed by conduct that isn't aligned with broad social norms. If I believe it's my duty to show up for a dinner date on time to the minute, I may feel shame for showing up five minutes late, even though that's perfectly acceptable socially and no one at the dinner cares. We all have an inner Arbiter of Right Conduct—we're all a society of two, at a minimum—and that judge's values may or may not be aligned with the cultural rules of the road.

A Useful Emotion. Though painful, shame is a useful emotion. Not always, but often. If I forget that Valentine's Day date, shame signals me that I've created a disconnect and prompts me to do what I can to make things right again. This probably means an apology, and it may mean other things such as a special gift or a declaration of intent to never, ever, miss Valentine's Day again.

If I feel shame, it means I care about the regard of others. It means I'm a healthy social animal. It means I want to do right by other people.

Not everyone feels shame. Those who don't are sociopaths, defined as "a person with a personality disorder manifesting itself in extreme antisocial attitudes and behavior and a lack of conscience." Feeling shame means you're not a sociopath and that's a good thing.

Which isn't to suggest that shame is always a positive emotion. There's nothing good about feeling ashamed because you're a gay man or a woman who loves sex. When you feel shame because you've been force-fed a disempowering cultural narrative, it becomes something to purge. Sometimes shame is warranted and sometimes it's not.

In either case, though, shame has value. It invites us to look more closely at what we're feeling and why. It may mean, as in the case of the Valentine's Day dinner, that you need to make amends. Or it may mean that the time has come to establish a more honoring and respectful connection with yourself and to hell with what other people say.

One hears talk these days that the bedroom should be a "shame-free zone." People who advocate this are essentially saying that it's fine to be totally comfortable with your sexual preferences and turn-ons. I agree that this is a good thing. If you're gay, be proud of it. Ditto if you're kinky or have politically incorrect sexual fantasies. There's an important proviso, though. What goes on in the bedroom isn't only about our relationship with ourself. It's also about our relationship with others, and here shame can be a healthy emotion. It's how we know there's been separation and it's what fuels the drive to re-connect.

The Experience of Shame

Having examined what shame is, let's look at what it looks and feels like.

Shame has a physical component. When we're ashamed, we flush, our neck and shoulder muscles go slack, and we're reluctant to make eye contact. Not only dogs look hangdog—people do, too, when they feel shame.

People can also have their own individual response to shame. If I find myself grinding my teeth, it tells me I'm feeling ashamed.

Shame also creates feelings of social isolation. You feel dropped into a pit of your own making and totally alone. You want to disappear.

In ancient times, the worst fate that could befall a person was to be sent into exile. It usually meant death because people couldn't make it on their own. Shame provides a sort of self-imposed preview of this experience—it's like pre-emptive exile. It's almost as if we've judged ourself, found ourself guilty, and imposed the appropriate punishment before the community can get around to it. *I'll do it myself, thank you.*

Children tend to think in black-and-white terms: 'I am bad,' not 'I behaved badly.' Shame can take us to that regressed place. The precipitating event is experienced as confirming an ancient, internalized story about the bad person we really are. *This proves I don't belong. This proves I'm not normal. This proves I'm unworthy.* Shame sends us on a high dive into the waters of self-loathing, which in turn can send up an entire cannonball of shame. A common next step in the sequence is to feel that a secret and humiliating truth has been revealed. *Not only did I behave unworthily, but now you know me for the unworthy person I really am!*

Shame can evoke other painful emotions, too. As children, we had zero shame resilience. The adult experience of shame can send us back to that panicky, helpless childhood sense of being in a nightmarish place with no way out. Same as it ever was, the monster has us in its grasp again.

Shame has this way of piling on. Some random event triggers the emotion, a biochemical cascade kicks in, and before you know it you're feeling separated and isolated from your peers, hopeless and helpless about yourself, and revealed to the world as the loser you really are. No longer are you the multi-faceted person you previously knew yourself to be. Shame reduces and defines you. Your name is now Shame.

Shame in the Bedroom

Shame when we're having sex is almost never a good thing. It creates separation, which is the exact opposite of what we want to do when we're in the bedroom, which is connect.

Shame inhibits communication along with connection. This is because, as we've seen, shame tends to render people mute. But people aren't only silenced because they *feel* shame. It also happens when they're concerned about *triggering* shame—in either direction. If I have a foot fetish, I might not mention it to my partner because I'm afraid their response may land as shaming. If I want more foreplay from my partner, I might not ask for it because I'm worried that it will land as a criticism and they'll feel ashamed.

A common complaint of heterosexual women is that they can't give sexual guidance to their men. Even if it's intended to be constructive, feedback of this sort often evokes feelings of shame because many men have internalized the cultural story that guys should know how to please their woman without any special guidance. Instinct and intuition rule, right? Which can only mean that when a woman speaks up, it means the man is screwing up. No other possible explanation!

Above, I wrote that shame is *almost* never a good thing. Why the qualifier? For two reasons. If she says, "Never, ever spank me" and you keep doing it, it's probably a good thing if at some point you feel shame. In addition, shame can be transmuted into a turn-on. We often eroticize things we find difficult as a way to gain mastery over them. If I'm ashamed of my need to be in control, I may enjoy being dominated sexually. If I'm ashamed of my inability to assert myself, I might get off on being a dominant.

And then there's the familiar female fantasy in which they don't really have a choice and are rewarded, not shamed, for letting go sexually. They're sex slaves on a pirate ship or on the receiving end of a gang-bang. When fantasies like these have power for women, it can be because it helps them process shameful feelings about their love of sex. They are granted permission to be lusty and promiscuous without being slutty because sluts *choose* to have sex and in their fantasy choice is denied them. Plus, no one could reasonably blame or shame them for giving themselves over to pleasure because, in contrast to normal society, where being sexually free and uninhibited is said to lose you the all-important protection of a man, here survival and sluttiness are aligned—terrible things might happen to you if you don't give your captors the full-slut response they're after.

Fantasies like these can be an emotionally healthy response to the sex-negative indignity of slut-shaming.*

Cultural and familial programming are frequent causes of sexual shame. Let's say that when you were a child, your father walked in on you while you were masturbating in your bedroom. Maybe he freaked out about it and shamed you because of all his unresolved shame from when he was a boy and his parents freaked out at him. Or maybe he ignored it, which isn't much better because it creates a culture of secrecy and silence and is also very shaming, albeit less directly.

There's a third way. Dad could have chosen to directly, lovingly and supportively address what he saw, a wise move that would have helped him heal his own shame and put an end to the negative cycle. How likely is that, though? It's the rare parent—and probably not yours—who's that self-aware. If you're like most people, you learned as a child that masturbation is something to hide, something to be ashamed of.

Now you're an adult. Is it any surprise that you hide your self-pleasuring from your partner? Or that, if your lover wants to watch you play with yourself, feelings of shame arise?

In addition to being handed stories about what constitutes shameful sexual behavior, we also get ones about what constitutes 'right' or 'good' sex. For instance, the conventional view has it that sex consists of foreplay leading to penetrative sex culminating in orgasm, ideally for both partners. This is how it's done—anything else is a deviation from the norm. While there's a compelling logic for this model—it's your basic mating sequence—it's overly

*** There can be other reasons for these fantasies as well such as the re-enactment of sexually traumatizing experiences. The same fantasy can mean different things for different people.**

technical and misses many of sex's wonderful rewards. Where in this narrative are the emotions? Where is the connection? The heart?

The highest purpose of sex is connection. You can have a great connection in the bedroom without following the conventional protocol, but it probably won't happen if you 'should' on yourself and don't give yourself permission to go where the dance takes you.

Let's say you're a man and can't get an erection. If you've bought into the conventional story line about good sex requiring penile penetration, you'll likely feel ashamed about your soft-off—and doubly ashamed if you also make your erectile dysfunction mean you're not a real man. But if you can embrace the view that great sex is ultimately about connection, then you can keep from turning your flagging member into a Flag of Shame and have a fabulous session. You can give your partner an orgasm orally. You can give them one manually. You can spin a fantasy while your partner self-pleasures. You can receive tons of pleasurable stimulation and even have an orgasm without being hard. There are all kinds of ways to have hot fun without a hard-on once you let go of expectations, limited sexual scripts and shame.

Another reason shame can arise is when one person says something their partner experiences as shaming. It may be intended to be shaming—or not. Sometimes a gentle request for a move adjustment ("a little faster, please") is all it takes for their partner to hear it as a commentary on their competence as a lover.

The trigger doesn't have to come from someone else. We all have voices in our head and some of them are critical. If I've decided I'm not a good kisser, I may find myself having to fend off feelings of shame when I'm locking lips with my partner, even if they're totally happy with my technique. (And of course, if they're not thrilled by it and they request a change in technique, my shame is compounded and can be devastating.)

So much shame. So many reasons for it. Is it any wonder that it shows up often in the bedroom?

Developing Shame Resilience

Shame doesn't have a cure. Feelings have a mind of their own and show up when they want to. But we can make it a lot less painful. We do this by developing shame resilience.

This is something we work on over time—it's an aspect of our personal growth curriculum.

This process has three components.

The first requires us to examine the stories we've taken in with our cultural mother's milk. Some we'll want to keep and others we'll choose to discard. If I'm gay, I'll want to exorcise any homophobic narratives I've internalized. If I'm a woman who really loves sex, I'll want to let go of any sex-negative stories I've bought into about female desire being bad.

Disempowering narratives are rarely erased overnight. Like vampires, they're adept at regaining their power and coming at you again and again. Keep at it, though, especially with the help of friends, and sooner or later they'll get that much-deserved stake in their heart.

Which brings me to the second part of the program. Find people you can talk to about your shame. Surface it in community with others.

As we've seen, shame silences and separates us. When we passively let this happen, we're giving shame power over us—we're giving it permission to burrow a hole deep in our soul. We don't have to surrender, though. When it comes to shame, resistance is definitely not futile—we have the power to exile shame rather than let it exile us.

We do this by going public with our shame, discreetly and appropriately. Just as silence empowers shame, speaking up disempowers it. Every time you share your shame with another person, you're declaring to the world, "I'm not ashamed of my shame. I'm okay with this aspect of who I am, okay enough to share it with someone else." And of course you're also declaring this to your shame. You're taking your shame into community and, in so doing, stripping it of its power to reduce and isolate you. *In yo' face, shame!*

In our culture, it's especially difficult for men to talk about their feelings. As boys, we have our feelings shamed out of us. We're told to suck it up and be a man. We're told to get tough. We're told to man up. As a result, when men slip into the shame loop, they often lack the skills to talk about it. No wonder, then, that so many men withdraw into their man cave and keep silent about this stuff! It's a subversive act—and I mean that in a good way—when men give their shame a voice, whether that means talking with someone else or journaling about it.

If you do choose to share with others, select your allies carefully. You don't want to be bringing your shame to someone who shames you for it. Choose friends who are real friends, who are wise and caring enough to want the best for you.

Another great option is support groups, whose express purpose is to help people be resilient in the face of a disempowering compulsion or narrative. Support groups are 'counter-communities,' self-organizing clusters of people who come together to free themselves from harmful attachments and embrace more empowering ones. While I don't know of any support groups that focus explicitly on shame, you'll have no trouble finding a group that supports its members to show up authentically—and that includes speaking up about their shame.

I'm also a big fan of therapy, both on your own and as a couple. When you work with a professional, you're seeing someone who's been trained not to shame. This is a good thing—and you'll also want to be discriminating in your choice of therapists. Just because someone has a degree doesn't make them a good therapist. If they haven't processed their own shame, there's a pretty good chance they'll project it onto others, including their patients. If your therapist says something that triggers your shame, pay close attention to what's going on. You may be getting triggered over nothing, but they may actually be shaming you.

The third part of the process is bodywork. Body and psyche are interconnected. If there's shame in your emotional body, it will show up in your physical body and vice-versa—the two reinforce each other. Massage and yoga are two of the many modalities that can help you release embodied shame. If you know how your shame expresses somatically, so much the better—you can focus your bodywork on those tensed-up jaw muscles, or wherever.

> *Find people you can talk to about your shame.*

When Shame Arises in the Bedroom

Developing shame resilience is a long-term project. Sometimes we'll do better at it, sometimes not so well. There will still be times when shame arises, and unless we're really skilled it can get pretty bad. Let's say Joe and Jill are playing in the bedroom and Joe can't get hard. Jill is sucking away and sucking away and getting no response from anything but her jaw, which is growing wearier by the moment. Joe feels ashamed about his 'lack of manliness' and it cuts deep because he has ongoing anxiety about how he stands with other men—this confirms his fear that he's a beta guy, or worse. Meanwhile Jill is feeling like a total failure because this is the third guy she's been with this year who's had erection problems, and isn't cocksucking supposed to deliver instant results? So she must be pretty bad at it, and while she's at it she's always hated how her breasts look, so that probably has something to do with it, too.

Shame, meet shame. We're not talking about personal growth now, we're talking about crisis management. What steps can the partners take to rescue themselves and each other?

Before anything else, they need to notice what they're feeling. They need to recognize the symptoms and say, if only to themselves, "Oh, I feel shame!" Self-awareness is the first step to getting out of the mire.

Next, they need to take action. A good place to start is with their physical response. When we feel shame, we tend to hold our breath, and when we do get around to breathing, it's shallow and tight. There's a double rationale for this. We feel less when we breathe less, so it's a way for us to numb our pain. In addition, when we get still, it's like we're going into hiding—it's got a whiff of self-imposed exile.

We can undermine this impulse by consciously taking deep, slow breaths. Doing this has a calming effect and enables us to keep from being totally bowled over by our shame.

Another way to keep shame at bay is by actively inviting it to go away. When people give speeches, negative thoughts sometimes arise. They're afraid they've lost their audience or fear they're losing their train of thought. An effective way to deal with this is by telling those negative thoughts, "Not now. I'm sorry, you'll have to go away." It's pretty much the same way you'd treat your child if they walked in on you while you were having sex: "Not now, I'm sorry, you'll have to go away."

You can treat shame like that intrusive child. You bring a protective curtain down around you and those shameful thoughts are, that's right, exiled. Firmly but not harshly, they're invited to go away.

Because shame loses its power when it's brought into the communal space, speaking up can help, especially if we're confident that our partner won't shame us if we do. It's not enough just to acknowledge how we're feeling, though—it's important to choose our words carefully. There's a world of difference between saying "I'm ashamed" and "I'm feeling shame." With the former, we're identifying our entire being with the negative feeling—we're saying our name is Shame. When we say "I'm feeling shame," we're acknowledging its presence without letting it colonize us.

No matter how ashamed you're feeling, the reality is that other things are going on, too. You're feeling hungry or thirsty, or you're wondering in a remote corner of your mind what your kids are up to, or you're noticing how sore your jaw is from all that cocksucking. Don't bury these aspects of yourself by using language imprecisely! Word-boundaries quarantine shame and keep it from metastasizing.

If you've tried these things and they haven't kept you from sinking into the pit, it's time for more drastic measures. Emotions are like weather systems. They come and go, and sometimes they hang around for too long, like a stationary low. We can shift this energy by changing our set and setting. Go for a walk. Jump up and down. Shake, shake, shake your booty. Make loud, funny, grunting sounds. Do yoga. Watch television, even! Which, though not often touted as a cure for anything, can do a pretty decent job of shifting you from low to neutral.

Don't just flee the room, though: Remember you're in community here. Explain to your partner what you're planning to do and why, and assure them you'll return when you're feeling back on your game. Although your shame may tell you otherwise, they have feelings too: You don't want to trigger feelings of abandonment in them by fleeing with no explanation. A good rule of thumb when you're feeling agitated is, minimize harm. Do what you can to maintain a good connection despite your upset.

There's a world of difference between saying "I'm ashamed" and "I'm feeling shame."

It may take a while to clear yourself of your shame energy—15 minutes, 30 minutes or more. Let time work its magic. Eventually the storm will pass and you can return to your partner, take a deep breath and start over.

Partners, what should you do if your partner plunges into shame? In a phrase: Validate and hold space. In a misguided attempt to make their partner feel better, people often say things like, "It's not a big deal," referring to what precipitated the shame. Unfortunately, this response doesn't shrink the shame—it shrinks the person instead. It can land like the person is saying, "You're overreacting," which translates into the invalidating "you shouldn't be feeling what you're feeling."

A far better approach is to acknowledge what you're witnessing: "You seem to be feeling a lot of shame." When you respond like this, you're gently and non-judgmentally inviting your partner to talk about their feelings.

Don't try to distract your partner, either. "*You think you're feeling shame? Let me tell you about the time when . . .* " Comments like will usually land like an encroachment on your partner's space, as if you're meddling and, again, denying them the right to have their feelings. Gentle support is the ticket here. Listen well, inquire tactfully, and hold them if they want to be held. (Ask first!)

Be the good parent.

* * *

The romantic myth, which is really a romantic fallacy, has it that you fall in love and live happily ever after. Love, all-powerful love, inoculates you against the bad stuff. It ensures that it never happens.

We have a similar myth about the bedroom. Sex is like a magic carpet ride. It unfolds without blips or blunders and sends you on a straight shot into ecstasy.

Uh, not where I come from. It's people who have sex and people are imperfect. Which makes their sex imperfect, too.

You develop shame resilience by becoming adept at dealing with shame when it arises rather than by going blithely along expecting things to go perfectly—and then freaking out when they don't. Although you may be assuming otherwise, 'sex masters' aren't perfect lovers. This is so for a simple reason: Like Santa Claus and the Easter bunny, the perfect lover doesn't exist. A true sex master is highly skilled at the sex stuff and at something else as well—they have systems in place for managing the emotional fallout that occurs when the erotic train goes off the rails.

Shame resilience is part of our emotional immune system. It keeps us from getting sick at heart in that special way we know as shame. It keeps early symptoms from blossoming into a raging shame flu. And it plays a hugely important role in helping us stay healthy, happy and connected in bed.

Learning to live with, listen to and heal shame isn't something that happens overnight. But each small improvement we make in our relationship to it brings more ease and pleasure to our sex lives and our connections with other people. That reward is well worth the effort.

SEXY SUMMARY

We don't talk about shame, but it crops up sometimes when we're having sex.

Shame isolates us and disrupts connection.

The best way to deal with this feeling is by developing shame resilience.

The three keys to developing shame resilience are: 1) exorcising shaming stories we've internalized, 2) sharing our feelings of shame with others, and 3) using bodywork to clear shameful feelings from our body.

If you go into a shame tailspin in the bedroom, take deep, slow breaths; speak up; and if necessary do what you have to do to clear the energy.

If it's your partner who goes into shame, listen well, inquire tactfully, and hold them if they want to be held. Be the good parent.

JESSICA O'REILLY *(Dr. Jess PhD) is a leading sex and relationship expert and author of the best-selling books, The New Sex Bible: The Complete Guide to Sexual Love and Hot Sex Tips, Tricks and Licks. She is the host of PlayboyTV's hit reality series, Swing, and facilitates couples' retreats around the world from the sunny Caribbean to the European countryside.*

Jess has worked directly with thousands of singles and couples and her advice reaches tens of millions across the globe. She is regularly featured by Cosmopolitan, Men's Fitness, Women's Health, The Huffington Post, City TV, Canada AM, CBC, ABC Spark, Playboy Radio and Breakfast Television, to name a few. She also engages hundreds of live audiences each year at a range of events including clinical conferences, professional development workshops, trade shows, fundraisers, community service groups, colleges/universities and corporate retreats.

Catch up with Jess on Twitter, Facebook & Instagram by following @ SexWithDrJess or check out her work online at SexWithDrJess.com.

NADINE THORNHILL *started her career in sex education as a part-time workshop facilitator in Ottawa, Ontario after twenty years working in theatre as an actor and playwright, She quickly developed a passion for learning and teaching others about sexuality. Her combined experience in theatre and sex education eventually led to a position as the Program Coordinator for Insight Theatre, an educational program for teens at Planned Parenthood. She also began her career as sexuality writer. Through her articles, advice column and blog, Nadine quickly became known for her friendly, relatable approach to sexual subject matter.*

In addition to her private sex-ed practice, Nadine is a member of the American Association of Sexuality Educators, Counsellors and Therapists as well as the Sexuality Information Council of Canada. She is currently completing her Doctor of Education in Human Sexuality, with a concentration on child and adolescent sexual development.

Nadine lives in Toronto, Ontario with her partner and their son. In her spare time she enjoys caterwauling at karaoke, eating good food and watching bad television.

Website: nadinethornhill.com

Facebook: facebook.com/nadine.thornhill

Twitter: @NadineThornhill

CHAPTER NINE

Keeping the Flame Alive

Carl Frankel in conversation with Jessica O'Reilly and Nadine Thornhill

EDITOR'S NOTE: ANY ROMANTIC RELATIONSHIPS LOSE THEIR SPARK over time. It's a pervasive problem: Reddit has about 20,000 members in its 'Dead Bedroom' subreddit. In this chapter, we bring together sex educators Nadine Thornhill and Jessica O'Reilly for a dialogue on how to deal with Dead Bedroom Syndrome.

Carl: Nadine, I understand that you have some personal experience with Dead Bedroom Syndrome.

Nadine: That's right. Much of what I've learned—and teach—comes from personal experience. I've been in the same relationship for 20 years and we've had a child for seven. Even before we became parents, there were ebbs and flows in our relationship. The first time things cooled off a lot, it was very alarming to me. I started doubting myself and the relationship. I kept asking myself why I wasn't feeling all that sexy energy that I had been feeling and believed I was supposed to feel. I now understand that it's very common in long-term relationships. I didn't at the time, though. I thought there was something wrong with me and us. I felt isolated in my situation and so did my partner. Some of our conversations got very fraught.

Jessica: Dead Bedroom Syndrome can be very painful.

Nadine: Yes—unsettling and upsetting. Suddenly I was opting to watch television with my partner rather than have sex. It would be the end of the day, I'd have been working and taking care of my child and doing all the other things I needed to do. Faced with a choice between sex and TV, I knew that if I watched Orange Is the New Black, I'd have a good time. I'd laugh, I'd cry, I'd have a fabulous evening. And if we had sex, we'd feel pressure, it would feel like work, and we couldn't be positive that it would end wonderfully—and if it didn't, we'd have to deal with doubts about ourselves and our relationship. So: On the one hand, a surefire pleasant evening. On the other, anxiety possibly leading to dejection. No wonder I chose television!

I was embarrassed by this. Even though I felt more deeply intimate with my partner than ever before, I believed that if your relationship was truly valid, it would be hot and heavy all the time—and it wasn't. Sexual desire came and went. This pattern went on for years. Whenever there was an ebb, I felt a lot of anxiety and this made things worse because we were putting pressure on ourselves to be sexual with each other in a way that wasn't congruent with what we were actually feeling. When we had sex, we both felt lots of pressure because we weren't just having sex, we were trying to validate our relationship.

Jessica: I suspect that many people who are dealing with Dead Bedroom Syndrome are thinking, 'I can relate.' I know that I still struggle with the fear that our sex life isn't as hot as it could be—or as hot as it should be. I've been with my partner for nearly fourteen years and I'm intensely attracted to him. Everything about him excites me from the way he speaks to the way he wraps his massive hands around my waist. But despite the undeniable attraction, I'm sometimes too lazy, tired, stressed or distracted to make a move. If he initiates, I'm game, but when the onus falls on me, I don't always act. And I always feel conflicted. After all, I'm a sexologist and that adds another layer of pressure. On one hand, I know I'll enjoy it if we get started, but on the other hand, I really love just being with him. I have to remind myself that sex is important to the relationship, but it isn't a bellwether of its success. Finding a balance between making sex a priority and allowing our sex life to arise naturally has been fundamental to alleviating the pressure and getting my needs met better.

Carl: So far, we've talked about how common and normal Dead Bedroom Syndrome is and how it's showed up in your relationships. Perhaps you can now discuss how to deal with this problem?

Jessica: I'll start. Broadly stated, there are two general approaches to dealing with Dead Bedroom Syndrome. The first is about attitude adjustments—doing inner work. The second bucket is programmatic. Not 'how can I change my perspective' so much as 'what actions can my partner and I take that will make things hotter between us?' While I believe that inner work is really important, and I definitely have recommendations for that area, I also believe that partners can choose to interact in ways that will help complement the inner work.

Carl: This is a great distinction. Inner Work, meet Programmatic! Let's discuss each in turn.

Attitude Adjustments

Nadine: Things began to turn around for me when I started re-writing my internal narratives about what these shifts in my relationship meant. Marty Klein's book *Sexual Intelligence* was transformative for me. One thing I learned from it is that the falling-in-love feeling we get is actually a biochemical cascade with a maximum shelf life of about four years. After that, those romantic feelings start to fade. What was happening to us wasn't unusual or a symptom of deep relationship problems. We weren't outliers—we were normal.

Carl: What else did you learn from Klein?

Nadine: That it's normal for our sexuality and sex drive to evolve over time. Our bodies change. Our hormones fluctuate. There's nothing 'wrong' with us if we have to re-visit what works for us sexually. Change comes with the territory—not just of relationships, but of life. Again: What we were experiencing was normal. Klein's book helped me be kinder to myself—less critical and more self-accepting. Instead of measuring my sex life against a false standard of what we 'should' be doing—so many times a week, how passionate and orgasmic—I authorized myself to be more connected to what my body was actually telling me. Once I was able to have a more honest, intimate conversation with myself, it also became easier to talk honestly with my partner about the reality of what we were experiencing.

Jessica: Performance pressure and manufactured cultural prescriptions can wreak havoc on an otherwise okay sex life. Not only is pressure antithetical to pleasure, but the pressure to perform according to some ridiculous cultural standard makes all of us question whether our sex lives are good enough. We don't need to seek cultural validation to tell us if we're happy. We simply need to look to ourselves.

I'm frequently asked how often the average couple has sex. While it's natural to wonder, this isn't a useful benchmark for measuring the quality of one's sex life. For one thing, it's a hard number to measure accurately. And more importantly, you should only be doing what feels good for you. Don't bother comparing yourself to averages and don't let cultural prescriptions interfere with your own estimations of sexual satisfaction. Lead your life, not some mythical other person's.

It's also important to remember that sex doesn't have to be mind-blowing every single time. The truth is that most of us don't have time for ecstasy on a Tuesday night after a long, hard day's work. Sometimes sex is just a release. Other times it's more about the connection and intimacy. Sometimes, you'll have trouble connecting and may just help one another to get off and ease the sexual tension, but this doesn't mean the relationship is failing. Even the best cooks burn a meal or overcook the pasta sometimes. The same can be said of the best lovers—we all have our off days and we need to lighten up and cut ourselves and our partners some slack.

Nadine: In addition to rewriting my story about what our relationship should be, I found myself re-visioning my notion of what was supposed to happen during our intimate time together. Klein's book was useful here, too. Instead of intending to have sex, we'd get together simply to be together and see what happened We'd commit to turning off the television and being focused on each other without feeling the need to 'get down.' If our time together got hot and heavy, great. If not, that was okay, too. It didn't mean our relationship was terrible. If all we did was cuddle, that was fine. Cuddling is great!

Carl: As I've talked with the sex masters of this book, it's become increasingly clear to me that sex isn't really about sex. Obviously, it's lovely if sex happens and even better if it's great. Beneath all that physical pleasure, though, the real reason we're getting together is to be present and intimate with another person—and sex can be an amazing way to achieve this. What you're saying appears to come from the same source.

Nadine: Yes.

Jessica: Culturally, we're hung up on quantity at the expense of quality. Sex is no exception. We insist on counting everything related to sex—number of partners, orgasms, frequency, time elapsed, organ length, size and of course, frequency. If we imagine applying this quantitative approach to other pleasurable acts, we can see how nonsensical this is. What if we ate food solely for the purpose of caloric consumption or visited art galleries with the goal of seeing as many pieces as possible? Pleasure isn't quantitative, it's qualitative, which means that once we shift our focus to quality over quantity, pleasure returns to the forefront.

Again, this is about shifting our narratives around sex. A useful first step in this direction is to ask yourself a simple question: What feelings do you want to experience through your sex life? Do you want—and this is not an exhaustive list—to feel connected? Loved? Cared for? Safe? Secure? Strong? Weak? Dominated? Submissive? Ecstatic? Excited? Once you connect sex with specific feelings (emotional and/or physical), it becomes easier to shift the emphasis to the quality as opposed to the frequency of the experience.

Nadine: Agreed—and we can achieve some of these feelings through intimate times with another person that doesn't include physical sex. Obviously, to deal completely effectively with Dead Bedroom Syndrome, it's not enough to have plenty of non-sexual intimate time together. You want to re-ignite your sexual connection. This is what the programmatic piece addresses. You want to create a context in which that program can flourish, though. Expanding your palette of 'okay activities,' of non-failures, is a great way to help create that favorable context. Less pressure—good!

Boundary Issues

Jessica: When we reframe the meaning and purpose of our intimate time together, what we're really doing is redefining our boundaries. We're expanding our notion of quality intimate time so it can include connecting without physical sex.

Nadine: This isn't the only boundary that warrants re-visiting. There's also the invisible but very real 'sex/no-sex' boundary—you know, the line between when you're being sexy or sexual with each other, and when you're not. These ways of being with each other tend not to overlap, and as you get deeper into a relationship, the not-sexy times start crowding out the sexy ones. As intimate partners, we can consciously choose to make this boundary more permeable by actively seeking out moments of connection, sensuality and sexuality. You can flirt, for instance. It may not be 30 minutes of epic flirting, but you can be erotically appreciative. If you think your partner's ass looks hot, you can say it, using PG language if your child's around and you think that's called for. You can give them a look that says, "I'm totally turned on by you right now." You can kiss.

Jessica: Yes. One of the most important elements of keeping the spark alive involves weaving eroticism throughout your relationship. I mean this in a practical sense, not a spiritual or mystical one. A brush of the thigh or a stolen glance can go a long way to keep the sexual energy flowing when you begin to live like roommates or siblings.

One of the biggest mistakes we make involves waiting to start foreplay until we're ready for sex. Foreplay is more effective when it starts hours, days or even weeks in advance. A little flirting, a few compliments, some warm skin-to-skin contact remind your partner that you're not just friends, roommates and/or co-parents. You're also lovers.

Focus on connecting during your intimate times together.

It's hard to flip a switch at the end of the day and become sexual after hours of work, cooking, cleaning, child-rearing and running errands. We need to be reminded of our sexuality throughout the day in order to be ready to turn it on in the evening. Partners can help each other do that without having it mean, "Now we're going to have sex."

Carl: Nadine, I assume that being a parent makes it more difficult to overcome Dead Bedroom Syndrome.

Nadine: It does make things more challenging. Realistically, if you're a parent, it's highly unlikely that your sex life is going to be what it was when you didn't have kids. If you are managing to have the same sex life as before, congratulations—you're a sexual prodigy. For most of us, we're not thinking sexually as much because our focus in on parenting. Our sleep is messed up. There are hormonal changes. Still, there's no law that says you can't be flirtatious or sexy with your partner when your child is around.

Carl: I can already hear people screeching about how you're corrupting your child. Tell me why you're not.

Nadine: We live in a sex-negative culture that tells us sex is inherently bad and corrupting. If you approach sex from that perspective, of course you should keep it away from children because if they see it, they're going to lose their innocence and become twisted. In fact, quite the opposite is true. Adolescents and young adults who have grown up in sexually healthy and expressive households report having higher levels of sexual satisfaction, and they also tend to have better sexual health outcomes—fewer infections, more consistent practicing of safer sex, more assertive communication skills, and so on. You're not going to turn your child into a depraved monster by being flirty or sexy when they're around.

Jessica: Nor are parents who are sexually expressive in front of their children paving the way for teenage promiscuity. Research confirms that early sexual health education that is comprehensive and addresses a range of topics does not hasten sexual activity. In fact, sometimes it delays sexual activity for teens!

Nadine: I know from being a parent that modeling is a really powerful way to teach children. They pick up more on what you do than on what you say. I want my son to see what consensual, pleasurable sexual communication looks like. I've worked with teens for years, and one of the biggest issues many of them have around sex is confusion about how to proceed. "I don't know how to talk to somebody about sex," or "I don't know how to tell somebody that I find them attractive without being gross about it." If you grow up seeing communications like this happen in a respectful, loving context, they becomes normal for you and you're better equipped to deal with these situations when they arise in your own life.

Something else that is really important for me because I'm raising a boy is that, by watching how I interact with my partner, he can see how boundaries are constantly shifting and being negotiated. Let's say my partner gives me a friendly slap on my ass or wraps his arms around me. Ninety percent of the time, that will be fine. Occasionally it won't be and I'll say so. It's really important for kids to see and understand that consent is always in play without its having to be heavy or a big deal. We don't have to sit down and have a super-serious conversation about it—it's just a natural part of our relationship. We also talk in front of our child about things like contraception and safer sex.

Carl: Where does the line cross from appropriate and acceptable sexual behavior to conduct that's over the line?

Nadine: In my workshops on this subject, I use the movie rating system. G, PG, PG-13, R and X. The 'R' is anything that's graphic. The definition of what this is will vary from person to person. Speaking for myself, I'm certainly not going to engage in any behavior in front of my child that might lead to an orgasm.

Carl: What borderline behaviors are okay and not okay?

Nadine: I think it's absolutely fine to enjoy passionate kissing or non-genital caressing in front of children. If the kids are old enough to occupy themselves safely for extended periods of time, I even think it's okay to let them know that you need a couple hours of privacy to be with your partner. Moves like caressing the breasts or touching the genitals would be off limits for me.

Carl: Any other thoughts about parenting and sex?

Nadine: Yes. There's an important distinction between sexual privacy and sexual secrecy. If my partner and I are having sex and our child walks in, it's totally appropriate to say, "This is private. Can you please leave and close the door behind you?" You don't want sex to be a secret, though. Kids will pick up on that and start to believe there's something shameful about sex. It steers them toward sex-negativity.

Carl: So far, we've identified possibly boundary adjustments in three areas—what a 'date' means, integrating more sensuality and sexiness into our normal routines, and bringing a more sex-positive environment into our parenting. Are there other boundary issues to look at?

Jessica: Yes. Some couples may find it useful to re-examine their boundaries with third parties around sex and intimacy. I'm not a proponent of any particular type of relationship because there is no one-size-fits-all approach to relationships. Still, I think it's a shame that as a culture we embrace monogamy without question.

Nadine: Polyamory—transparent sexual or intimate relationships with people other than your primary partner—can be a valid option for some couples. Sometimes people have differing sex drives or specific needs that their partner doesn't want to meet. Clearly, non-monogamy isn't for everyone, but some couples find that it works for them. Sometimes, in fact, the freshness of an outside relationship rekindles the fire at home! I'm not advocating polyamory. I am advocating being open-minded in terms of considering non-traditional alternatives to monogamy.

Jessica: Monogamy isn't easy—just look at infidelity rates! But non-monogamy isn't easy, either. Alternatives like swinging and polyamory take a lot of work. There's also a middle ground between the two, which I call 'Monogamy 2.0.' The partners are sexually exclusive with one another, but there's more acceptance of the fact that one or both partners may want to be sexual with other people. Monogamy 2.0 says yes to this reality rather than prohibiting it emotionally. It might involve having a self-pleasuring fantasy about a third person and inviting your partner to join you when you're ready for some real-life company. It might involve flirting with others and using the juice of that 'innocent' flirtation to stoke the fires when you're with your partner later that evening. Or you might push your sexual boundaries alongside your partner, for instance by attending a sex party together with the agreement that you'll only watch. Out-of-the-box experiences like these can bring you closer as you talk about your feelings, boundaries and fears in advance, offer support and reassurance during the experience and debrief in the afterglow.

Nadine: There's a larger point here. Dead Bedroom Syndrome happens because people get into a routine in their lives and with each other. Novelty, trying something different, is a way to disrupt this pattern and bring freshness and newness back into their lives. By shifting from the known to the unknown, by moving into a domain that's more about learning and exploration than doing the same old same old, we re-light our own fire—and that's a crucial first step to re-lighting the fire of our relationship.

Carl: Are there other mental or 'attitudinal' keys to overcoming Dead Bedroom Syndrome?

Nadine: Yes—take responsibility for your own sexual gratification. In long-term relationships, we start believing that it's our partner's responsibility to get us off. A lot of people have this notion that you shouldn't masturbate when you're in a long-term relationship—or if you do, you should do it secretly so your partner doesn't know about it. Problematic beliefs are packed into this behavior, like self-pleasuring is wrong when you're in a relationship or that your partner has failed you if you want to play with yourself. I'm a strong believer in making self-pleasuring part of your regular sex life, including intimate times with your partner.

For me personally, it's been really helpful to integrate masturbation into my partnered sex. Sometimes my partner will be touching me in a certain way and I'll be able to say, "Uh, no, that used to work, but it's not working anymore." There are also times when I'll say to him, "I'm just going to go in there for a second. Be here and you can watch and you can still be touching, but I need to touch myself for a bit and see what's happening down there."

Jessica: When we settle into a sexual relationship, we learn our lover's hot spots and sure-fire buttons. This makes sex easier and more pleasurable.

However, as we become familiar with our lover's unique sexual responses, we often stop exploring. This is unfortunate because, over time, how we experience pleasure shifts. It's constantly evolving. It's great to be in discovery together.

Nadine: When we integrate self-pleasuring into our relationship, both on our own and with our partner, it's empowering, it's restorative—and it can also be a great way to play together.

Carl: Speaking of no secrets, what about porn?

Nadine: Personally, I'm okay with my partner consuming porn. I watch porn, too. Sometimes we watch together, sometimes separately. There are certain kinds of pornography that he likes but I don't, but I'm not inclined to deny him that pleasure. I don't have a competitive relationship with porn, but I understand that everyone's different in this regard.

Jessica: Porn is ubiquitous. We've experienced a cultural and generational shift in which pornography is accessible and widely consumed. Twelve percent of all websites are porn-related and 25% of all Internet searches are for adult content, so we cannot talk about sex without talking about porn.

The good news is that there are now so many genres of porn available that whatever your fancy, you can probably find it for free online. Porn has the potential to reignite your interest in sex, generate new, meaningful conversations about fantasies and boundaries, and spark new and exciting shared interests for couples.

On the flip side, porn can take a toll on relationships and sexual identity if you use mainstream porn (the type produced primarily for men by men) as a tool of education. Porn is not education—it's entertainment. Comparing yourselves to porn stars is unrealistic and expecting your real experiences to look like their staged theatrical performances is equally impractical.

If you're tempted to try out porn as a couple, I suggest that you seek out couples' porn and watch it with no expectations if it's your first time. You may find yourselves tearing one another's clothes off, having a good giggle, or nodding off in boredom. Whatever your reaction, rest assured that you're perfectly normal.

As for the possibility of watching porn without your partner while you masturbate, I certainly don't consider this cheating. Ideally, you can be transparent with your partner and considerate of their feelings.

Nadine: The larger point isn't about porn or self-pleasuring. It's that, when you're in a long-term partnership, it's empowering for both you and your relationship when you take responsibility for your own sexual gratification.

An Rx for Dead Bedroom Syndrome

Carl: There seems to be a gray area between 'attitude and boundary adjustments' and specific programmatic shifts. For instance, if you change your attitude around self-pleasuring, your behavior will change, too. But there would also seem to be actions you can undertake independently of rewriting the stories in your head. Yes?

Jessica: Absolutely. We've already identified some of them, like starting foreplay outside the bedroom and making it part of your daily routine. There are other things you can do, too. One is to emphasize non-sexual touch. Physical affection can deepen your bond, lower stress levels, improve sleep patterns, elevate mood, lower blood pressure and strengthen your immune system. Also, express desire. Show your lover that you want him or her as opposed to expressing a desire for sex itself. Most people don't want to feel like they're a part of your weekly or monthly sexual tune-up. They want to feel like a sexy beast that you just can't wait to have sex with.

Carl: Anything else?

Jessica: Yes—lots. Speaking of sexy beasts—treat your partner like a piece of meat. When we first meet, attraction is at the forefront of our thoughts as we wonder about our love interest's naked body and sexual personality. Once we get to know one another, we stop looking at each other like animals. We tend to see respect and consideration on the one hand, and animal desire on the other, as mutually exclusive. This contributes to Dead Bedroom Syndrome. The next time your partner irks you with one of their annoying daily habits, choose to think of them as a piece of meat. Think of their butt, their breasts, their hips, their hands, their hips—whatever inspires you sexually. Instead of letting the resentment build, replace it with animal lust for the piece of meat that exists beneath their clothing.

Carl: How politically incorrect!

Jessica: The sexiest things often are. Speaking of which, here's another tip—talk dirty. When you do this, you're tapping into your most intense fantasies and bringing them to life in words. And since fantasy is often hotter than reality, crawling into your partner's dirty mind can be enormously helpful in firing up that familiar long-time relationship.

Carl: What else?

Nadine: Explore and experiment with your own body. A lot of us have techniques for masturbating that are familiar and may be very reliable in terms of producing an orgasm or releasing sexual tension. Try touching yourself in different places and in different ways, not necessarily with the goal of getting off, but to find out how your body responds. You may discover new paths to pleasure and you can share that knowledge with your partner.

Jessica: Also, allow yourself to feel sexual. Fantasize. Sharing your fantasies with your lover may seem intimidating at first, but once you start you'll be hooked, as the experience can further cement your bond. The mere act of talking about a fantasy (even with no intention of living it out in real life) can be arousing and lead to hot intimate interactions.

Allowing yourself to be sexual can include giving yourself permission to be turned on by other people. Sexual desire is fluid, so it's healthy to be attracted to a range of bodies and personalities. While many of us suppress our desires and fantasies due to cultural prescriptions of monogamy, fantasizing about other people is a safe way to broaden our sexual horizons and face this repression head-on. When your inner life is juicy, your relationship with your partner is likely to get juicier, too.

Carl: Give me more—I'm still not satisfied.

Jessica: Believe it or not—go out on double dates. According to a study from Wayne State University, hanging out with other couples can help to reignite the spark and increase feelings of passion within a relationship.

Last but not least, spend time apart. Absence makes the heart grow fonder—and the libido swell, too. If you spend too much time together, your appeal can be dulled by all that routine. Share parts of your life, but keep some components separate to maintain the novelty of passionate love.

Nadine: These are great suggestions—and the fact remains that Dead Bedroom Syndrome can be very challenging. It's a sort of entropy—we have to push against it constantly. So there's another piece to this—compassion.

When things aren't all you might wish for, have compassion for your partner and compassion for yourself.

Carl: Compassion for yourself—that's the hard part.

Nadine: I actually got the compassion piece from my partner. Our two best friends were moving in together and asked for advice about how to navigate their new life together. My partner said, "There are going to be times when you get on each other's nerves. When you have that moment of irritation, always remember that they love you and weren't doing this to try and piss you off."

Jessica: Yes! Not only are we too hard on others, we're also too hard on ourselves. If you're the type of person who will seek help through therapy or self-help books like this one, you probably put a lot of pressure on yourself. Letting go of some of this pressure can work wonders for your sex life. Know that simply by virtue of being willing to read a sex book, you're already ahead of 99 percent of the general population.

So, yes, be kind to yourself.

SEXY SUMMARY

- Examine your narratives around what's normal in a long-term relationship.
- Take responsibility for your own sexual gratification.
- Interject novelty into your relationship.
- Re-examine your boundaries around self-pleasuring, porn and possibly your definition of fidelity.
- Give yourself permission to be (appropriately) sexual in front of your children.
- Flirt! Touch!
- Embrace your 'inner sexy.' Fantasize. Talk dirty with your partner. View them (in a good way) as a 'piece of meat.'
- Be compassionate towards yourself and your partner.

Dubbed by her peers as the "approachable pervert," **EVE MINAX** *is a pleasure artist who delights in proliferating carnal knowledge. A domina, urban Tantrika and Bondassage practitioner, she is a certified Sex Educator and the lead staff instructor at the Cleo Dubois Academy of SM Arts. She is a frequent presenter at sexuality conferences, academic forums, and sex-positive community venues.*

Minax holds an MA in Gender/Sexuality Studies. She was the West Coast coordinator for the Leather Archives and Museum Roadshow. She is an advisor on the Research and Advisory Committee of CARAS (Community-Academic Consortium for Research on Alternative Sexualities) and a Board member of TASHRA (The Alternative Sexuality Health Resource Alliance). She has many projects currently in the works, including classes, performances and publications.

To learn more: EveMinax.com.

CHAPTER TEN

Eroticizing Safer Sex

by Eve Minax & Carl Frankel

FOR MOST PEOPLE, ANY CONVERSATION ABOUT 'SAFE SEX'—OR, worse still, 'safer sex'—is inherently depressing. The terms make a melancholy statement about the times we live in. They tell us we have to shackle our desire.

Responsible people understand that since the advent of HIV and other sexually transmitted infections (STI's), we often need to use protective barriers like condoms, dental dams and gloves. It's hard not to see this as a turn-off that leaves us longing for the time, not so long ago, when sex was about fun and freedom and not at all ominous.

Safer sex—aargh.

This would seem to make it my task in this chapter to reduce the turn-off factor of safer sex as much as possible. Eve your damage control specialist here, making lemonade out of lemons.

I don't see my assignment this way, though. Instead of viewing safer sex as an unfortunate necessity whose negatives need to be minimized, why not view it as an opportunity that, if creatively engaged, can make our intimate life sexier and richer than it could be otherwise?

Safer sex—the opportunity!

I'm not surprised if this sounds like a stretch. How can barriers possibly enhance sexual pleasure? But they can. Believe me, they can. Not only can we neutralize the negative impacts of protective barriers, we can turn them into a positive.

Defining 'Sex'

Let's begin by defining our terms, starting with what we mean by 'sex.' This is important because it will help us understand how protective barriers can increase our pleasure.

In 1998, when accused of having engaged in non-intercourse fun and games with Monica Lewinsky, including getting blow jobs and watching her insert a cigar into her vagina, then-President Bill Clinton said famously, "I did not have sex with that woman." Well, Bill, actually you did. For me, sex is any activity that, done without protection, puts you or your partner at risk of getting an STI. When Monica wrapped her mouth around the presidential penis, she put herself at risk of contracting human papilloma virus (HPV), chlamydia, gonorrhea and HIV.

And that cigar? Here, I'd argue that they weren't having sex because neither was at risk of contracting an STI. They were definitely being sexual with each other, though—we can probably all agree that when a man watches a woman masturbate with a cigar, it's qualitatively different from watching a football game.

It may seem like I'm splitting hairs here. For Hillary as well as all those Republicans who went in howling for the kill, both acts constituted adulterous bad behavior. The man was cheating on his wife. Enough said, right? Not quite. For our purposes if not the wife's and politicians', the distinction between 'having sex' and 'being sexual' is important. It defines the difference between sex play that is risky and sex play that isn't.

Defining 'Safer Sex'

Now let's consider what we mean by 'safer sex.' This one's straightforward: It's about reducing risk in our sexual encounters. How do we do that? First and most obviously, by using protective barriers—latex or nitrile gloves for hand play, condoms and dental dams for oral sex, and condoms for vaginal and anal penetration.

There's another crucially important piece of the puzzle—communication. To practice safer sex, partners need to negotiate what they will and won't do. Clarity and precision are essential here. If Joe and Jill agree to use condoms, that's the beginning, not the end, of the conversation. Will they be using them for oral sex as well as vaginal intercourse? How about anal sex—is that on or off the table? (Or the bed, or wherever.) And what about dental dams, which are the equivalent of condoms for cunnilingus? If the only protective barrier mentioned is condoms, this invites a misunderstanding. Jill might assume the term includes dental dams because she views them as the female version of a

Safer Sex Hierarchy of Risk

NOT RISKY ('BEING SEXUAL')
Massage; Hugging; Fantasy; Voyeurism; Exhibitionism; Masturbation; Non-shared sex toys; Dry Kissing; Body-to-Body Dry Rubbing; Phone Sex; Watching Erotic Films; Reading Erotic Literature.

POSSIBLY RISKY
Wet Kissing; Shared Hand & Genital Contact with a Barrier; Oral-Genital Sex or Oral-Anal with a Barrier; Fisting with a Barrier; Genital Sex with a Barrier.

PROBABLY RISKY
Shared Hand, Finger & Genital Contact with open cuts, wounds or sores; Oral Sex without a Barrier.

VERY RISKY
Oral Sex without a Barrier during Menstruation; Male or Female Ejaculate in the Mouth, Vagina or Anus; Oral-Anal Sex without a Barrier; Fisting without a Barrier; Shared Sex Toys without a Barrier; Shared Needles; Sucking Breasts of a Lactating Woman; Vaginal or Anal Sex without a Barrier.

Reprinted with Permission: Sheri Winston's Center for the Intimate Arts

condom, while Joe might assume he's free to lap and lick away unobstructed because their 'contract' was silent about Saran Wrap. If you don't get clear on this sort of thing, you're asking for trouble.

There's a time to have these conversations, and it's not when things are hot and heavy. The brain goes on vacation when the blood rushes south. When you're highly aroused, it can be difficult to form coherent sentences, much less have elaborate conversations about what protective barriers will be used when. That romantic dinner is the time to have these discussions, not when things are on fire in the bedroom.

No safer-sex conversation can cover everything, though. Reality being what it is, you may need to discuss something when you're in the throes of passion. At times like this, a safe word can help. Fewer syllables: better.

Safer sex is ultimately about caring—for yourself and your partner. It's about being respectful and considerate. Let your conversations reflect this—and bear in mind that people also communicate without words. If I smack your bottom and you push it toward me, you're telling me you liked it and

YOUR GUIDE TO PROTECTIVE BARRIERS					
	HAND	MOUTH	ANUS	VULVA	PENIS
HAND	None	None	Glove	Glove	Glove
MOUTH	None	None	Oral Dam	Oral Dam	Condom
ANUS	Glove	Oral Dam	N/A	N/A	Condom
VULVA	Glove	Oral Dam	N/A	Oral Dam	Condom
PENIS	Glove	Condom	Condom	Condom	Condom

Reprinted with Permission: Sexuality.org

want more. On a similar but negative note, if I try to penetrate you without first having a safer sex conversation, I'm telling you I don't care about you or your well-being. Safer-sex talks may seem like an onerous obligation, but they're a lot more desirable than a sexual encounter that leaves you feeling shabbily treated.

Fire Up Your Imagination

Sex isn't just a physical act. It also inhabits what more than one person has called the body's most erogenous organ—the mind. When Bill and Monica shared that cigar, they were turning themselves and each other on mostly with their minds. He wasn't only being aroused by the fact that she was inserting a phallus-shaped object into her vagina. It was also that she was choosing to behave so sluttily for him. Similarly, it was hot for her to know that she was arousing this man seated at his desk—all the more so because he happened to be the most powerful person in the world. The cigar was their launch pad into a mirrored world where they were feeding off each other's perception of the other. They were playing mind games with each other for their mutual pleasure.

The mind is hardwired for arousal. A cigar can do it and so can lots of other things. I'm a professional dominant and in my off hours, I have a submissive who serves me (voluntarily, of course). When I see her doing my dishes, I get turned on. To a visitor, it may seem like my submissive is doing a menial chore. For me, it's sexual behavior.

Here's my point: Our minds can eroticize anything. If we don't, it's only because we tell it not to. I believe this is because we're afraid of what will happen if we give our sexual imagination free rein. It's true that sex is a supremely powerful energy—and it's also true that most of us suppress it unnecessarily. Our fears notwithstanding, just about everyone can do a fine job of controlling their lust even if they don't try to squash it. I have a vivid sexual imagination, and I'm also highly socialized and not a source of public depravity. While not everyone fantasizes about firemen in chicken suits, I'm just like everyone else (or almost everyone else) in my ability to behave appropriately when the situation requires it.

As discussed in Megan Andelloux's chapter (*Fantasy, Role Play and Communication*), a liberated erotic imagination is a fine thing. And it's relevant to this discussion because the more we can free up our erotic imagination, the hotter our safer sex will be.

Cultivate a Positive Attitude

As a professional dominant, over the years I've become expert at turning people on with just our psychological interactions (and some visual stimulation, too). This, in turn, has taught me an enormous amount about how to make encounters super-sexy.

We all have the potential to be amazingly sexy—if we let ourselves be. We've got our imagination, we've got our words, and we've got our desire—and by that I mean not only our desire to have sex, but also our desire to take and be taken, to dominate and be dominated. These are our tools for generating arousal. Use them skillfully and that condom stops being a bummer.

Before any of that, though, you may need an attitude adjustment. If you're bummed at the prospect of using protective barriers, you'll be less able to have hot sex. When you're being sexy, you're engaging Eros, the creative life force. Negative thoughts interfere with your ability to make this connection. If you're feeling annoyed, irritated or sulky, it will be reflected in how you feel and what you do, and it'll be less fun for you and your partner.

The mind isn't only our most important erogenous zone. It's also how we make sense of our daily experiences. When such-and-such happened, it was a good thing. When something else happened, it was bad. We construct these stories around just about everything, including safer sex. 'Protective barriers make sex less sexy' isn't true or false. It's a story, and the thing about stories is they can be changed. 'Protective barriers make sex possible' is as true as 'protective barriers make sex less sexy.' It's also a lot more positive. As a first step toward eroticizing safer sex, I encourage people to start thinking positively about protective barriers. It's better to view them as a gateway, not a wall—to cultivate an attitude that says, 'In this age of STIs, protective barriers are what make that hot date possible.'

People can also help their partner cultivate a positive attitude about protective barriers. A great time to flip that switch is during your safer-sex negotiation:

Cultivate a positive attitude about protective barriers.

JILL: *I'm glad we're having this safe sex conversation. What kind of sexual activities are you hoping to have with me?*

JACK: *Well, everything, actually.*

JILL: *Everything? Including anal sex?*

JACK *(salivating heavily): Oh yeah!*

JILL: *I find you really attractive, so I'll let you do me in the ass—but only if you wear a condom.*

JACK: *C'mon, Jill. I hate condoms.*

JILL: *But you love ass-fucking, right?*

JACK: *Oh yeah. It's my all-time favorite.*

JILL: *Well, then, imagine this: I'm on my knees and elbows. You slide your cock in my ass. I'm so tight—and you slowly open me up. I love it so much. I surrender so good when I get it in the ass.*

(Jack listens silently. A fleck of spittle appears on his lip.)

JILL: *I'm getting hot just thinking about it. (Pause.) Now about that condom . . . .*

JACK: *Sure. Whatever. Just let me at you!*

From impediment to opportunity, in one juicy conversation.

Integrate, Integrate, Integrate

Now you've made that attitude adjustment—what's next? Integrate those hot and yummy barriers into your foreplay. If the guy you're with isn't thrilled at the prospect of wearing a condom, his feelings will probably change if you apply it with your mouth. (It's even sexier if you can do it without laughing.) For your part, you may find that condom literally distasteful—and it's true, ice cream does taste better. There are ways to make the experience more pleasant, though. Coconut oil is a great and tasty lube, and it makes a condom go down more easily.

Which will make you go down more easily, too.

(Don't use coconut oil with a latex barrier, though. The two are incompatible. If you're going to use coconut oil, I recommend polyurethane condoms.)

While it takes some effort to make condoms sexy, that's not the case with dental dams, which I can view with no challenge whatsoever as a great sex toy. Recently someone was complaining to me about dental dams. "Who would want to use them?" she asked. "They just get in the way." My response was,

"No, they're wonderful." My answer came from the heart. First you arouse the pussy by caressing it, with or without gloves depending on what you've negotiated. Here, too, great lube helps. Once the pussy is all swollen and juicy, you put the dam on and squish it around. It feels totally amazing, even better than a tongue in some ways. Dental dams produce their own special, wonderful sensation. It's like you've got a mythic sea creature down there, doing weird sea-creature things to your tender bits.

We can even turn protective barriers into a turn-on just by seeing them. I buy black latex gloves by the case. The sight of them turns me on and I'm further aroused when I pull them on. It's a simple act, but it's packed with significance—it speaks to all the pleasure I've gotten in the past and to all the pleasure I'll soon be giving and receiving. My partners get turned on by this, too. They know what those gloves mean to me—this is the mind-mirroring principle at work—and they also know what my pulling them on says about what's in store for them. My, how I love my black latex gloves! They're both a safer-sex barrier and a heart-thumping turn-on for me and my partners.

Integrate barriers into the pleasure process.

The Power of Arousal

Here's another strategy: Distract your partner so he or she doesn't notice or care about the fact that you're using protective barriers. How do you do this? By making them crazy with desire. If it's a condom that's the issue, make his cock so hard and play with it so long that its happy owner barely notices that it's somehow gotten sheathed in a condom. Arousal is an altered state—this is not just a metaphor, it's a physiological fact. If you alter a person's awareness dramatically enough—if you take them deep enough into their arousal trance—details like gloves or a condom will barely be noticed, much less seen as a problem.

More broadly, remember these three words when dealing with the protective-barrier challenge: Foreplay, foreplay, foreplay. That's the secret ingredient for getting to such a high level of arousal that gloves, condoms and dental dams shrink to insignificance. You'd think this would be obvious, but it's not. Culturally, foreplay is sadly misunderstood. The average sex act, including foreplay, lasts under ten minutes, yet women need up to 45 minutes of foreplay to become fully aroused. Women are getting the shaft—and not in a good way.

We live in a hurry-up society that favors fast food and, it seems, fast sex. While I'm all for the occasional quickie, slower is usually better and a lot slower is better yet. It's juicier, deeper and more fun. If I have one bit of advice for men about their lovemaking, it's this: Slow down! Women appreciate a man with a slow hand—and a slow everything.

Partly because we have such hurry-up notions about sex, our cultural understandings of arousal and orgasm are badly distorted. When the foreplay is brief and the arousal level modest, the level of pleasure will be modest, too. When the arousal level is allowed to build slowly over time, it opens the door to ecstatic and orgasmic experiences that are off the bell curve. Women can have orgasms that last for hours. Men can have non-ejaculatory orgasms that go on and on. Once you ascend to a level of arousal that makes these sorts of experiences possible, those protective barriers will be a pebble, not a boulder. Barely noticeable.

Your foreplay doesn't have to be risky. Energy sex (see Chapter 15) is a great way to increase your arousal, and you can do it in a fully-clothed, no-risk way. You can also increase each other's turn-on before you get to the bedroom. You can sext or have phone sex. You can watch porn together. You can kiss and nibble and whisper sweet somethings to each other throughout the day. You can also get outrageous: When was the last time you wore a sex toy to your favorite restaurant? The best foreplay doesn't last ten minutes or even an hour. It starts in the morning and lasts all day.

Once you're in bed, there are all kinds of ways to 'use your sexy.' Here are some suggestions:

- Sexual fantasy. "Did you know that these gloves put out little pleasure pulses like tiny electric charges?" "Did you know that these are special condoms with female arousal hormones in them? When I put it on you, I get so turned on I almost come!"
- Sexual promise (of pleasures to come). "Once this condom is on, you're going to get the fucking of your life."
- Sexual appreciation. "I love how your cock/pussy looks. It's beautiful and it turns me on."
- Sexual sharing. "I love how it feels when you [fill in the blank].
- Sexual inquiry. "Do you like it when I do ... this? How about this?"
- Sexual teasing. "Would you like it if I licked you like this?" "Imagine what it'll feel like once that condom is on and you slide your cock into me."
- Sexual display. "Do you like how . . . this . . . looks?"

- Sexual power exchange. "Crawl over here with that dental dam/condom in your mouth." "Say 'Thank you, Master/Mistress' when I put my hand on your cock/pussy."

Note that words are involved in all these examples. Although silence can be sexy (has anyone out there ever used a ball gag?), as a general rule silence is a turn-off and talking is a turn-on (if it's on subject, of course).* At the end of the day, sex is about connecting with another person and that's what words do—they tell the other person what's going on in our heart, our mind and our lewd imagination.

We all come off the assembly line endowed with lots of sexy. Forget how society says you should be. Use your sexy. Use your words, your body and your imagination to make you and your partner tropically hot. Do that and you'll find yourself feeling much more positive—or, at a minimum, neutral—about protective barriers.

Dentists have a trick for minimizing the pain of being injected with Novocain. They take a chunk of cheek between two fingers and waggle the skin as they slip the needle in. The commotion distracts the brain so that it barely registers the needle's sting. Arousal works similarly—and it's much more fun. If the partners are feeling dizzy with ecstasy on Planet Turn-On, they'll barely notice the 'sting' of protective barriers.

Living the Life Erotic

When we embrace our sexy self, we're tapping into Eros, the most powerful force on the planet. It's not only the procreative force, it's also the creative force—the source of all things generative. Every time we want to produce something new, whether it's a baby, a work of art or a screaming orgasm, that's Eros doing its thing. It's the best high ever and we don't need drugs to get there.

How sexy can you make your life? How sexy can you be? I'm not suggesting you dress to attract wolf whistles. I'm inviting you to get sexy on the inside, to tap into one of the most primal forces on the planet. All organic matter comes into life; all organic matters grows; all organic matter dies. This process is life's essence, and it's driven by the generative principle. By Eros. By tapping into your own erotic nature, you're tapping into your most creative, passionate and alive self.

*** Making sound is also a great turn-on. It lets your partner how much you're enjoying the experience, and it has the added benefit of serving as guidance. Sound means, "Keep doing this!" An extended silence means, "Please try something else."**

I love to sail. Being out on the water turns me on: I actually get a bit juicy. I think of it as 'erotic lite'—while it's not as directly sexual as when I pull on my black latex gloves, it does have a sexual component. What if we were to actively seek out the erotic in all we do? I'm not suggesting that we should all start thinking like young teenage boys: I'm not proposing that we get juvenile or tawdry. I'm actually suggesting the opposite, that we seek out the erotic so we can celebrate it for what it is—something true and beautiful and divine.

I actively seek out the erotic in every corner of my life. It's my chosen path to living fully. I speak from experience when I say that the more you can live erotically, the less troublesome protective barriers will be. Why? Because, when you're living in your pleasure, you're less likely to make mountains out of molehills.

Or gloves. Or condoms.

Like life, safer sex is what you make of it.

At the end of the day, it's your choice. You can make safer sex a really annoying problem. Or a non-issue. Or a wonderful way to play.

SEXY SUMMARY

IT'S IRRESPONSIBLE and inconsiderate not to practice safer sex.

IT'S POSSIBLE TO TRANSFORM condoms, gloves and other forms of safer-sex protection into ways to actually have more fun.

USE YOUR SEXUAL IMAGINATION! It's a fabulous way to turn on your turn-on.

NEVER UNDERESTIMATE the importance of arousal. Lots of it.

MAKE A PRACTICE out of eroticizing life.

MEGAN ANDELLOUX *is the founder and director of The Center for Sexual Pleasure and Health (The CSPH), a 501(c)3 organization dedicated to reducing sexual shame, challenging misinformation and advancing the field of sexuality. She is a board-certified ACS (American College of Sexologists) Clinical Sexologist, an AASECT (American Association of Sex Educators, Counselors and Therapists) certified Sexuality Educator and a recently appointed ISSWSH (International Society For The Study Of Women's Sexual Health) Fellow. Her innovative education programs, writing, social media presence and ambitious speaking schedule have helped make her one of America's most recognized and sought-after experts in the growing field of sexual pleasure and health.*

She is an in-demand lecturer at universities and medical institutions nationwide and has delivered her dynamic programs at more than 190 institutions of higher education and 50 medical establishments since 2009. Ms. Andelloux is also an Adjunct Instructor at the Brown University Medical School and the Brown University Pediatrics Residency Program.

She is frequently called on by TV networks for her insights and commentary, including CNN, NPR, MSNBC, Fox, and ABC as well as radio and print media. She has been labeled by the press as "The Princess of Pleasure," and "The Sex Ed Warrior Queen." The industry also recognizes her leadership in the field of sexuality. Ms. Andelloux was presented with the 2012 First Tracks Award for Innovation in Sexology by Honest Exchange.

Author of Hot and Fast: Sexy, Spontaneous Quickies for Passionate Orgasms *(Amorata Press, 2012), Ms. Andelloux has also written timely consumer feature stories, industry trend reports, and journal articles for the education and research communities. In 2011 she published* Sexual Health Education and Policy in Medical Schools: The Importance of Incorporating Basic Human Rights into Medical Education and Training, *which led to her involvement in the first Summit of Medical School Sexual Health Initiative, held in Minneapolis the following year.*

She can be found on social media platforms under HiOhMegan or TheCSPH. To learn more, visit TheCsph.org or OhMegan.com.

CHAPTER ELEVEN

Fantasy, Role Play and Communication

by Megan Andelloux & Carl Frankel

I'LL START WITH THREE BASIC QUESTIONS.

What's the relationship between fantasy and role play?

Why do the two matter?

And finally, what do they have to do with communication?

Fantasy is what goes on inside our minds. We all have fantasies—lots of them!—and most aren't sexual. If someone cuts us off while we're driving, we may fantasize about rear-ending them or running them off the road. We don't do these things, of course. They stay fantasies.

We also have sexual fantasies. In many ways, they're the same as our non-erotic fantasies. We're simply imagining what we'd like to do. But they're also different. They're charged, and not just with sexual energy. Many erotic fantasies take us out of our comfort zone to places where we start asking ourselves, "Yikes, is this really me? Is it okay to desire this? Is there something wrong with me?" Fantasies can challenge our self-image in a way even angry non-erotic fantasies don't. If I fantasize about running some jerk off the road, I don't ask myself, 'Does that make me weird? Am I a bad person?' I just have my vindictive little fantasy and get on with things. But if I fantasize about something sexually edgy and taboo, that can easily make me uncomfortable in skin and soul. We have a lot of fear related to our sexually-themed fantasies, although they're essentially no different from our non-erotic ones.

One reason our sexual fantasies are so charged is that they sometimes transgress cultural norms. If I've been raised in a homophobic society and have homosexual fantasies, that can cause me to feel socially disqualified, as if my membership card should be revoked. Cultural norms are powerful and, for that reason, oppressive. It can be difficult for people to feel okay about themselves if their culture tells them they shouldn't.

This is why it's so important for us to get in touch with our fantasies—it empowers us. What goes on in our sexual minds is okay, no matter what it is. There are no mind crimes: We have a right to be who we are. If we want to lead our lives as free, empowered individuals, we must learn to accept ourselves, including those aspects of ourselves that run counter to what society favors. At the end of the day, if we spend our lives not exploring beyond what's socially sanctioned, we're doing ourselves a disservice. We're limiting our freedom and our capacity for celebration and delight. While getting in touch with our fantasies can and does add juice to our sex lives, that's ultimately a secondary benefit. More fundamentally, it's an exercise in self-empowerment. In personal liberation.

There's an ongoing tension between, on the one hand, our cultural and societal boundaries and, on the other, our longing to celebrate and delight in who we are as individuals, never mind how we're supposed to be. In this contest, I stand squarely on the side of the individual. Freedom matters. A lot.

This does not mean freedom to *do* anything. Just because a fantasy turns us on doesn't make it okay to act on it. Although I do believe that there should be no boundaries around our sexual imaginations, I also believe we need very clear boundaries at the point of intersection where interior fantasy meets actual behavior. If you're going to pursue a fantasy in the real world, it can only be with a consenting adult. Anything else is grossly abusive and totally unacceptable. Just because I'm totally libertarian about what goes on inside our heads doesn't mean I believe anything goes in the space where bodies interact with bodies. Everything I say about total freedom inside our minds has a flip side: There are powerful constraints on what we may do in the world. It is a moral (and legal) crime of the first order to impose our sexual will on non-consenting beings.

There are no mind crimes.

I'm a rape survivor and so this isn't an abstraction. I feel very strongly about this.

There's quite a contrast here. Is it really possible to be totally uninhibited in the exploration of your fantasies while also exercising rigorous control relative to how you translate those fantasies into behavior? It's like having one faucet wide open and the adjacent one shut tight.

For the vast majority of people, this doesn't even begin to approach being a problem. Most people know the difference between right and wrong and aren't psychopaths. If you do happen to be in the small minority of people who have difficulty managing the boundary between the imagination and action, please get help. Personally, I don't believe there's much if any value in trying to censor your imagination. The work you need to do is around managing your behavior, not your fantasies.

Erotic fantasy, then, refers to what turns us on sexually. It inhabits the imagination and may or may not be something we would or could do in the physical world. If I get off on the idea of having sex with ten-foot-tall extraterrestrials from the Pleiades, that's a fine fantasy but I probably won't actually be able to make it happen, not even with the help of craigslist.

But I might be able to find someone who would pretend they were the hot extraterrestrial of my dreams. This would be role play—acting out a fantasy. Thus, not all fantasies involve role play, but all role play involves fantasy. Role play invokes an age-old template—children playing pretend. "Let's play pirates!" Only this time it's "Let's play pirates—and I'll be the hunky captain and you be the gorgeous prisoner!" Role play is X-rated playtime for grown-ups.

Communication merits a place in the title of this chapter for two reasons. First, because you can't have really great sexual interactions without equally great communication. The familiar porn image of a guy banging away while she rolls her eyes in mock ecstasy—that's poor communication. They're not telling each other what's working for them or what might work better. How often in porn do you hear "A little to the left" or "Rock, don't pump"? As for the guys, they often act as if they've wearing a ball gag even when they're not. How often do you hear male porn actors telling their partner what's making them so hot? "I love it when you trace the edges of your breasts with your fingers!" "You're so gorgeous when you're deep into your desire like you are now!" Communication before, during and, yes, *after* sex is enormously important.

It's easy to fall into the trap of thinking that great sex is about getting off, or getting off a lot, but that's only part of the story—and really the lesser part. Having great sex is more fundamentally about connecting with another person. Not just their body parts—the whole person. It's about laughing. It's about delighting. It's about screwing up as well as screwing. "Remember that time we fell off the bed together?" Sometimes the biggest foul-ups are the things we remember and delight in most. Great sex is about sharing pleasure and delight. If you're deadly serious when you're having sex—if you never smile or giggle—you're sort of missing the point. Fabulous sex is about being intensely human with another person. It's a really fun exploration, and that involves, by definition, lots of communication. Being silent behind the wall of your anxious thoughts ("Am I doing it right? Is my cellulite a turn-off?") doesn't enhance your experience . . . or your partner's. It creates separation.

The second reason communication is really important is because it can be very difficult to talk about our fantasies. What turns us on sexually is very private and personal. It's easy for people to go through the motions and move their bodies in the way magazines tell them to or in imitation of what they see on the Internet. But, to actually recognize the uniquely personal fantasies that arouse us and then to share them with another person puts us in a vulnerable position. For all we know, they may laugh at us or turn away disgusted. One of the greatest obstacles to having an amazing time in bed is being afraid of what people might think of us. That makes us afraid to talk. The remedy for this is to get out of our own way and share the fantasies that make us really hot.

This remedy involves a three-step process.

First, we have to discover what turns us on. This isn't always as easy as it sounds. If I view myself as totally heterosexual, homosexual fantasies may be very threatening to me. Yet at the same time, if I can somehow muster the courage to go there, I might find that they're a total turn-on. Just the fact that I'm "breaking the law"—the law of my internalized permission system—can feed my arousal. So can the freedom I discover in exploring uncharted erotic territory. Honoring and celebrating every aspect of oneself, especially those that have been consigned like Cinderella to the cellar, is always a turn-on.

Second, we have to learn to be okay with our fantasies. This isn't always easy, either. If Jill has been raised to be the proverbial "good girl" and finds herself fantasizing about gang bangs, that can be difficult for her to accept. If her fantasies have her totally objectifying her partner, that may be challenging if she's been told all her life that she should be sensitive to other people's needs.

This tension crops us fairly frequently in feminist circles, where the cultural rhetoric has it that having fantasies about being spanked or raped is wrong and inappropriate—a personal shortcoming, really—because you're playing into the patriarchal guilt system—your desire to be dominated or humiliated reflects centuries of male domination. But some staunch feminists have these fantasies anyway. This kind of cognitive dissonance can be emotionally troubling but the sexual imagination doesn't care. It's stubborn—it wants what it wants and refuses to get 'should' on. I don't believe our politics have a place in the boudoir. The bedroom should be where we free ourselves, not operate under constraints.

The larger point, though, remains: For a whole host of reasons, it can be very challenging for people to be okay with their sexual fantasies.

The third and final step in our process is sharing our fantasies. This is another big challenge. Until I discuss my turn-on with you, I can't know how you'll respond. You may find my fantasies kinky, deviant or—worse still—disgusting. I may find myself labeled a pervert by you. That'll be tough on my self-esteem and, quite possibly, on our relationship.

The risks of communicating about our sexual desires aren't limited only to our fantasies. If I like to have sex with lots of partners, including ones I'm not especially close to, and if I share that fact with someone I want to be transparent with, I may find myself labeled a sex addict when I was hoping to be seen as a free spirit.

And, it's not only sex that has risks. Communicating about sex does, too . . . and yet we have to do it.

Discovering What Turns Us On

So here we are in this uncharted territory called Our Sexual Fantasies. How do we find out what they are?

I'm a big fan of making it a fun research project. With all the Internet porn that's out there, it's pretty easy to explore what turns us on and what doesn't. There are also books with great erotic fantasies, such as those by Nancy Friday and Allison Tyler.

It's reasonable to wonder why we need to do this special exploring. Many of us have been masturbating since puberty and our imaginations are usually chipping in. Doesn't this mean we know what turns us on? Not necessarily. What worked at puberty may still get us off, but it's probably not the only possibility. When we stick to our tried-and-true fantasies, we're limiting ourselves. It's as if we're driving on a highway through a forest. We can see the trees on either side of the road, but we have no idea what might await us if we parked and went hiking. If we go deep, we often find that what turns us on is transgressive and a bit shocking. Our hottest fantasies aren't safe, not because we're at risk of inappropriately taking them out into the world, but because they challenge our sense of who we are.

We shouldn't let that stop us. We are who we are, and that includes these forbidden flowers. There's not a standard sexual way to behave, nor is there a standard sexual way to get turned on. I'll say it again: We are free individuals with a total and unconditional right to our sexual fantasies. So why not discover and celebrate them?

So, now you've done some research and found something, maybe in a book or on the Internet, that's kind of intriguing. What next? Incorporate it into masturbation time or into a sexual encounter with another person. You don't need to actually share the fantasy—if that's going to happen, save it for later. But just let your imagination go with the fantasy and check out how it feels. Does it enhance your erotic experience? Does it work for you? Playing with new sexual fantasies is like trying on a different style of clothing and finding how it looks on you.

It might feel a bit uncomfortable the first couple of times you play with the fantasy, as if the outfit doesn't quite fit. That's understandable: This is edgy territory you're stepping into. Be kind to yourself. Give yourself permission to take this hike into the woods. Better yet, applaud yourself for it. This isn't only an exercise in sexual arousal, it's also an exercise in self-empowerment.

Don't fret about your sexual fantasies. They're no more meaningful than that time you imagined keying someone's car (and didn't do it). Honor and play with your fantasies. See where they take you.

Communicating Your Erotic Fantasies

As we've seen, sharing our fantasies can be pretty scary, especially if they're not of the plain-vanilla, socially-accepted variety. Yet you've got to take the plunge if you want to share those fantasies with a sexual partner. The best outcome, of course, is to get an enthusiastically positive response from your partner so that you end up incorporating these fantasies into your shared sex play, whether through role play ("This time, you be the Martian!") or narration ("And then the three guys tied me up …"). While you can't count on that happening if you do share, you can be sure it won't happen if you don't.

I recommend approaching this difficult subject gently and indirectly. Don't bring it up while sharing a romantic candlelight dinner and don't bring it up while naked, either. Broadly stated, you'll get one of three responses: Enthusiastic support and approval, rejection and disapproval, or—and this one happens frequently!—an awkward silence. Learning that your partner has a wild and bizarre fantasy can be a lot to take in. You can sometimes get a long silence as the person tries to absorb this new information. Unfortunately, that silence is open to a lot of interpretations, including "Oh my God, he (or she) is trying to figure out how to not tell me how disgusting I am!" All in all, it's best to avoid situations that lend themselves to eye-to-eye discomfort. Structure the setting so your partner can have their reaction without feeling the need to respond to you right away.

One way to do this is by sharing your fantasy during a car ride, which is one of those situations where you can't spend extended amounts of time gazing into each other's eyes, unless you want to end up in a ditch. Let's say your partner is driving and you start chatting about something you saw on TV, or some celebrity who you heard is into something kinky, and then you drop a line into the conversation like, "I've been thinking about that activity and it sounds kind of intriguing. What do you think about that?" And then you look out the window, and your partner continues to drive, and eventually he or she will respond. Or not.

Riding in a car isn't your only option. You can also do it while you're working alongside each other, maybe while doing the dishes or weeding the garden. Whatever the specifics, the general principle remains the same. Broach the subject gently. Make it easy for it not to get heavy quickly. Set it up so there's not a big charge attached to it.

If you and your partner are into technology, that's another option. You might want to create a blog of images that you find sexy or arousing. You can make the blog private so only you and people you invite specially can see it. Tumblr is a great vehicle for posting your blog and also for finding images. It's got a huge selection, everything from kittens to porn. Photos are a great way to communicate about your fantasies because finding the right words can be challenging. But pictures tell all.

Here, too, the advantage is that you and the person you're sharing your fantasies with get to have separate experiences. They'll probably visit the blog on their own and thus have the opportunity to have their own reaction without having to deal right away with how to respond to you.

Tumblr blogs are a great dating strategy, too. If you send a person to your erotic-fantasy blog, it can be quite a turn-on for you both, especially if you're just getting to know each other. There's anticipation—"How will he or she respond?"—and surprise—"Wow, he or she is into that!" These are great arousal feeders.

One last point about communicating your erotic fantasies: Do it with pride. How you launch the conversation will often dictate how it goes. If your tone is sheepish and embarrassed, the person you're sharing with will pick up on that energy and be inclined to assume there's something in your fantasy to be ashamed about. Even if you're feeling a bit nervous, try to communicate with confidence. A dash of 'fake it till you make it' may be required: That's okay. Better to fake it a bit and end up with what you want than to be authentically insecure and end up with a communication fiasco. Your tone and attitude go a long way toward determining the response you'll get. If you project that you feel just fine about your fantasies, you're likelier to get a thumbs-up coming back at you.

There is a middle ground here. If you're feeling nervous about something, it's fine to say "I'm a bit anxious about raising this subject." That's just being authentic. But then, once you do get around to the actual discussion, be authentically in your self-respect. You've owned up to your feelings—now don't 'leak.'

Now we come to the flip side of this conversation. You've been on the receiving end of your partner's communication about their sexual fantasies, and they want to try them out with you. If their fantasy matches yours, no problem—you're off to the erotic races together. But what if there isn't a match? What if your reaction is indifference or disgust?

There are two basic principles to keep in mind here. The first is that there are no bad fantasies. Whatever you may just have heard, don't respond with anything along the lines of "Ew, that's gross!" You'll be doing yourself and your partner a service—your partner because you're protecting their feelings, and yourself because you're aligning yourself with the crucial principle that it's okay to be who you are—and that applies to you as much as to your partner. The likelier you are to go "Ew!" about someone else's fantasy, the likelier you are to do it to yourself.

Plus, that's probably the last time they'll ever share a risky fantasy with you.

Second, negotiate, negotiate, negotiate. Let's say your partner wants to try what is euphemistically known as 'water sports' . . . and less elegantly as 'piss play.' It wasn't easy for him or her to share, but somehow they managed, and now here you are with a proposition: Will you pee on your partner? Let's also assume this is over your line and not something you can imagine doing. None of this makes it okay for you to denigrate your partner or to abort the conversation with an abrupt "No way that'll ever happen!" Ideally, you'll respond respectfully and embark on a creative quest for a middle ground that works for both of you.

I think of this as the pizza approach to erotic problem-solving. Most people don't like the same type of pizza. Some people like olives and hate pepperoni, while for others it's the opposite. So how do people who are dining together select a pizza? By getting olives on one side and pepperoni on the other. In the case of our water-sport example, maybe you could help your partner find piss-porn. You could narrate a peeing fantasy while they masturbate. You could put hot water in a turkey baster and squirt it on them because that way they'd get the peed-on sensation without your having to do any actual peeing. Or—and this will be too much for many people—you could open up the relationship so they can find a pee-play partner.

The basic governing principle is this: Just because I'm not into something myself doesn't mean I can't support it in my partner.

It sometimes helps to unpack your "Ew" and discover the underlying reasons for your turn-off. In our current example, maybe you'll find that it's not the prospect of peeing on your partner that upsets you, it's the thought of wetting the bed! So maybe doing it in the shower, or covering the bed with waterproof pads, will do the trick instead.

A tolerant attitude and creative problem-solving are the keys to a healthy response.

Doing Role Play Right

This header is intentionally ironic. "Doing role play right" suggests there's a script to be followed and that's not the case, except in this one sense: Before anything else, role play is play. You "do role play right" by having fun.

Before you start, you'll want to communicate what you have in mind. You'll want to get clear about boundaries—what is and isn't okay—and you may want to agree on a safe word, a single word that communicates 'Stop what you're doing right now and back off.' It's best to have the safe word not be "stop" because mock-begging the person to stop is often part of the game. A word that's unlikely to make its way into your sex play is a better choice, like maybe 'rutabaga.' (Or something less silly.)

> *Be respectful and tolerant of your partner's fantasies. If they're over your line, try to find a mutually acceptable middle ground.*

Once you begin, you're doing an improvisation. The whole point about improv is that you're making it up as you go along. You're not feeding off a line-by-line script. You'll probably want to have a general set-up ("I'm the pirate and you're my captive"), but beyond that you'll be spontaneously inventing it as you go along. Just like kids. (Or, in this case, Captain Kidd.)

The first rule of improv is to always work with what your partner's doing . . . to say "Yes!" Don't negate it. If your partner says, "What a beautiful day!" don't say, "No, it's raining." That's deflationary—it kills the energy. Instead, say "Yes, and see over there? That looks like rainclouds coming in!" The same principle applies to sexual role play. Never negate your partner's contribution. Find a way to say "Yes!" and use it as a springboard to take you to the next point in the game.

Inevitably, screw-ups will happen. You're tying up your captivating captive and it's taking you forever to make the knot. You're spanking her because she was very, very bad and suddenly she farts. Go with what happens—remember, you're in an improv, not following a script. Who knows, maybe she farted on purpose and wants to see how you'll respond! Or maybe it was inadvertent. Either way, maybe a round of fart-training is in order!

If you need to re-group and start over, that's okay, too. Giggling is great: Giggling means you're having fun. Whatever you do, don't take it too seriously. You're not taking a test, you're playing a game.

One final piece of advice: Don't hurry. People tend to rush when they're feeling nervous. That's why inexperienced public speakers often talk too fast when they're giving a speech. So slow things down. Be patient. Let the game unfold in the fullness of time. You don't have to be doing, doing, doing all the time. Stillness can be hot, and so can going slowly. Burlesque is sexy precisely because it's deliberate. If you speeded it up—the woman comes on stage and ten seconds later she's naked—it wouldn't be sexy anymore. A slow burn is hot. So are teasing and anticipation.

Going slowly can be especially difficult for guys, especially younger ones, who often want to get their cock into the nearest available orifice as quickly as possible. This is totally understandable but often not the path to the greatest good time for both partners. My advice: Relax, take your time, and have fun.

* * *

It takes courage to share aspects of ourselves that transgress our own or society's norms. In its small way, it's heroic. Even if you have an icky response to your partner's out-there fantasy—and icky responses do happen; emotions have a mind of their own—I encourage you to remember how brave they're being. Meet their heroism with admiration or, at a minimum, respect.

Free your mind by saying "Yes!" to your fantasies wherever they may go. Free your heart by saying "Yes!" to your partner's fantasies even if you're not going to act them out. Fantasy and role play are wonderful personal-growth opportunities if you embrace them in that spirit.

SEXY SUMMARY

THERE ARE NO MIND CRIMES. Celebrate who you are! Go boldly where none have gone before.

BE RESPECTFUL of other people's fantasies. When you broach the subject of your own sexual fantasies, create space. Avoid situations where you're staring into each other's eyes.

WHEN YOU BROACH THE SUBJECT of your sexual fantasies, create space. Avoid situations where you're staring into each other's eyes.

IF YOU DON'T SEE TOTALLY EYE-TO-EYE about a given fantasy, be creative in exploring what might work for you both. Negotiate your way to a, um, happy ending.

HAVE FUN WITH YOUR FANTASIES and with the people you play with. (Giggling is encouraged … but optional.)

Advanced Skills and Special Treats

PATRICIA TAYLOR, Ph.D., *is the leading teacher of Expanded Orgasm in the world. Her studies in this field—extending back more than twenty years—inform her media appearances, two published books, a full-length sex education video, and countless popular classes and playshops. Patricia's website is ExpandedLovemaking.com.*

She recently released her programs, The Seduction Trilogy (seductiontrilogy.com) and Expand Her Orgasm Tonight: The 21 Day program for Partners (expandherorgasmtonight.com), a downloadable home study course for couples. She has hosted more 120 interviews of experts, writers, and extraordinary practitioners in the field of enlightened sexuality on her podcast, Expanded Lovemaking: Sex, Love and Consciousness.

Her books include the 1997 relationship masterpiece, The Enchantment of Opposites: How to Create Great Relationships, *and the bestselling 2002 classic,* Expanded Orgasm: Soar to Ecstasy at Your Lover's Every Touch. *Expanded Orgasm has sold over 25,000 copies to date. Expanded Orgasm has just been released in its second edition as of January, 2014.*

Her explicit DVD, Expand Her Orgasm Tonight, *demonstrates a woman in an expanded orgasmic state for over 30 minutes.*

Her studies are drawn from many sources, including bio-neural sexuality, More University, the Human Awareness Institute, hypnosis and Tantra. She is a California Certified Sexological Bodyworker. Yet, her most extensive experience stems from working directly with others and from her own ongoing rigorous practice of frequent extended, ecstatic Expanded Orgasms.

Dr. Taylor earned her Ph.D in Transpersonal Psychology in 2000 with the groundbreaking dissertation, "Expanded Orgasm as a Pathway to the Transcendence of Consciousness." You can download portions of this dissertation at scribd.com by searching "Expanded Orgasm" and Patricia Taylor.

CHAPTER TWELVE

Expanded Female Orgasm

by Patricia Taylor, Ph.D. & Carl Frankel

When I was younger, I had a near-death experience. It started out as a really scary event that wound up becoming an amazingly blissful experience. I went into the white light described by so many people.

These events caught me totally by surprise and changed my life forever. I had been working as a money manager on Wall Street. I was making lots of money and was a success by worldly standards. After my near-death experience, my job didn't have much meaning for me anymore. I started looking for pursuits that felt more aligned with the very different person I'd become. I became a student of Tantra. Along the way, someone said to me, "You really ought to try extended orgasm. I think you'll like it." I gave it a try and not only did I like it, it brought me back to a state very much like the one I'd been in during my near-death experience. It took me into a space that felt much bigger, more profound and more beautiful than my normal reality and led me to develop a fusion of extended orgasm and Tantra, which I called 'expanded orgasm.'

While expanded orgasm is a physically amazing experience, that's not why I became a student and ultimately a teacher of it. It's also a profound spiritual experience. It takes me out of myself and provides me with a deep sense of purpose and meaning.

Spiritual growth isn't the only reason to do expanded orgasm, of course.

If you're in a long-term partnership, it's a wonderful way to keep the relationship juicy. Entropy is the usual trajectory for relationships, no matter how much the partners love each other. We get used to each other, we get irritated with each other, we turn into each other's sibling—for a host of reasons, we shut down. We need something special to counteract all this negative momentum—some sort of positive force that brings joy, ecstasy and expanded awareness into our life. Expanded orgasm is a great way to do this. I've been married for over two decades and one of the main reasons our relationship is still going strong is because of our expanded orgasm practice. It takes us out of mundane reality to a place of profounder connection.

If you're just starting to date someone, expanded orgasm is a great way to create a memorable impression. Dating is a marketplace. When you can come and come and come, it makes you really popular—I can testify to this from experience! It gives you—a Wall Street term here—a competitive advantage.

It's also a way to shuck off all the mixed information—and misinformation—our culture feeds us about sex. If the only magazine you ever read were *Cosmopolitan*, you'd conclude that everyone has great sex and it's really easy to blow his mind with your virtuoso skills ("47 Ways To Make Him Want More!"). If *Redbook* were your sole source of information, you'd decide that relationships are chronically empty and in need of drastic intervention. Neither of these narratives is true, of course. The reality is more complicated.

Amidst—and in part because of—all these competing narratives, many people don't have truly fulfilling sex lives. A lot of other things get in the way, too. There are all the negative stories we carry around in our head ("My [fill in the body part] is ugly," "If I really let go, it'll mean I'm a slut"). There's cultural misinformation, much of it courtesy of porn (pounding is better, women love having men squirt cum all over their face). There's ignorance about the body and how to get it *really* turned on. There's the personal experience of trauma and abuse.

Expanded orgasm cleans out all these closets. It takes you into the Now and shows you up close and personal how amazing sex can be. This is one reason why it's such a fabulous personal empowerment practice. Part of this process involves developing and enhancing your ability to better distinguish your own authentic experience from the stories you've internalized about how things 'are' or are 'supposed to be.' Expanded orgasm lands squarely on the side of the real you, the authentic you, the you who has a right to experience amazing ecstasy based on the only script that really matters. The one that's written by your body, mind, heart and spirit.

Defining Expanded Orgasm

Before going further, let's get clear about what expanded orgasm means.

It's something both men and women can experience.

It's a *process*, a sequence of actions that brings a person into an *altered state* of blissful expansion and flow. The more you engage the process, the more skilled you'll become at switching into the realm of expanded orgasm.

My focus in this chapter is primarily on expanded orgasm for *women*, though men are equally capable of experiencing expanded orgasms.

Let's look at the conceptual foundations of conventional and expanded orgasms, bearing in mind that even though I'll be talking about women's orgasm, the experience is available to men, too. We usually think of orgasm as a climax, a peak. You come, then you come down. Expanded orgasm isn't a mountain peak, it's an entire mountain range. Once you start coming, your orgasms can continue for an hour or more. (Much more.) There will be peaks and valleys inside that high, but the entire journey is orgasmic.

Expanded orgasm is also less localized than the conventional genital orgasm—it's felt throughout the body. It is also usually experienced emotionally as well as physically. Body and mind no longer feel separate, but part of a larger self that includes your whole being, your play partner (if you have one), and ultimately the entire world. Expanded orgasm is to regular orgasm as a 16-course meal is to a simple dinner.

The foundations of expanded orgasm are *attention* and *connection*. Whether the circumstances are solo or partnered, the receiver is lavished with love. If it's a solo date, you act as your own best lover. If it's a partnered date, your companion brings the love—and so do you. There are technical aspects to expanded orgasm, but it's not just about technical competence. One of our most basic human needs is to be on the receiving end of a loving person's undivided attention. Expanded orgasm sessions deliver this experience.

I recommend practicing—and enjoying—expanded orgasm outside of your usual partnered lovemaking. This is easily achieved by setting up intentional practice dates. This way, you can experience expanded orgasms as their own separate activity.

That said, once it's relatively easy for you to go into the expanded orgasm state, there's no reason not to integrate it into all the aspects of your sex life. More pleasure: Better! And more orgasms are better, too.

If You're Orgasmically Challenged

If you have difficulty achieving orgasm, you're not alone. According to some studies, 50-75% of women don't come from vaginal intercourse without clitoral stimulation and 10% have yet to experience their first orgasm. Which raises an obvious question: Can anyone practice expanded orgasm, or is it limited to women who are already orgasmically proficient? Can ski bunnies go out on these slopes or must you have black-diamond skills?

My answer is unequivocal: It's for any and all women. Whether you've never had an orgasm or can 'think yourself off' (which is possible!), expanded orgasm can be a great practice. At a minimum, it can help you become more orgasmic.

That said, it's also true that you've got to crawl before you can walk. If you've never had an orgasm, don't expect your sessions to send you on an hours-long orgasmic ride. But carving out quality time for focused attention and connection in an erotic context will help you become more orgasmically proficient. It's a great practice regardless of your orgasmic level.

Foreplay, Expanded Orgasm-Style

For purposes of this discussion, let's assume your expanded orgasm session will be with a partner, not solo. (Let solo be an option for another time.)

One person is the receiver and the other is the giver.

An expanded orgasm session is a powerful ritual and it requires a strong container. This has two elements, physical and emotional. Givers, as the facilitator of the expanded orgasm session, it's your job to be your partner's caretaker. You want her to feel totally safe and taken care of.

One way to do this is by checking in ahead of the session. Giver, how are you feeling? How is the receiver feeling? Are there any time constraints your partner should know about? What about physical issues? Is there anything new or different you or your partner would like to try? If you're still getting to know each other physically, discuss foreplay requirements and other essential information such as how much lube she likes to use. While it's true that, as a general principle, women need more foreplay than men (much of it non-genital) to get fully aroused, it's also the case that expanded orgasm sessions have their own rules.

> ***As best you can, clear your minds before the session begins.***

I first studied extended orgasm with Victor Baranco and his teachers at a very alternative educational institution called More University. The approach I learned there teaches you to play with a woman's mind way in advance of a date. But once the physical connection starts, you are taught to go straight to the clitoris. It worked for me then and still does—and many other women find it works for them, too.

Don't assume anything here, givers. Check in with your partner. If she wants you to take your sweet time getting to her genitals, indulge her. If she's fine with your starting off with her vulva, then lube up your fingers and get going. There's no official 'right way' to proceed, only what works for her.

I also encourage givers to prepare the physical space for the session. Silence the cell phones. Pick the dirty clothes off the floor. Make sure the temperature's right. Set up the bed, complete with pillows (you'll want lots of them), lubricant, toys and a 'puddle pad' if your partner is an ejaculator. It's all a way of telling your receiver, "This is your time. You can count on me to take care of you. The only thing you've got to do is surrender into your bliss.

I'll handle everything else."

I can't stress the importance of this enough. To go into expanded orgasm, most women need to feel safe. They need to feel held—figuratively, if not literally. Givers, you have a lot of power here. You can facilitate this and you can also undermine it. Ideally, you'll show up as her protector. Her guardian. Anything short of that and she may feel the need to stay vigilant, which will block her from surrendering fully to the experience.

Givers, think of the pre-hands-on, 'setting the stage' portion of the date as mission-critical foreplay.

There are also your internal environments to consider. Here, the responsibility falls primarily on the giver (although the receiver can help out if she is generous and caring and thinks with enlightened self-interest). Had a tough day? Leave your unhappiness at the door. Get as clear, present and centered as you can. Take a walk. Meditate. Do Zumba. Do whatever it takes to get that negative or distracted energy out of your body. It will only get in the way.

How To Be a Great 'Session' Musician

An expanded orgasm session can last an hour or more. You'll want to be comfortable, very comfortable. Giver, this means resting up against a backjack or the bed's headboard with a bent knee. Receiver, have your legs open with one sliding under, or over, your partner's knee, depending on what's most comfortable. Use as many pillows as you need for support. A lot of us have aches and pains—you'll want to minimize them.

So now we're ready to get started. For purposes of this discussion, let's assume the receiver is fine with going directly to genital contact. A good opening move is to play with the labia. You can stroke them. You can massage them, that is, stroke them more deeply. You can open and spread them. You can roll them between your thumb and forefinger.

Another great move is stroking the length of the vulva on either side of the central opening, up and down, up and down, as if you were petting a cat. (It's not called the pussy for nothing!) If you press down so you're reaching below the surface, you'll be stimulating the vestibular bulbs, an important and often-overlooked piece of female erectile equipment.

Eventually, and perhaps sooner than later, you'll want to start playing with her clitoris, which is usually Action Central for expanded orgasm sessions. You can initially access the clit *through* the clitoral hood and simply press down, or press and pulse. You can squeeze it (gently!) between your thumb and forefinger. You can rub it gently, going over the top. You can circle it in a clockwise or counter-clockwise direction. You can focus on one particular area: Many women find the 1:30-2:00 zone to be especially delightful. If this isn't her hot spot, have her show you how and where she wants to be touched.

You have a lot of options here. Whichever you choose, I encourage you to experiment with using the pads, not the tips, of your fingers. Be sensual. Cultivate a mood of luxuriousness—lavish her with positive, highly-focused attention. Do your best to be centered, too. The best touch comes from deep inside you and transmits to deep inside her. It's not just finger to clit, it's heart-to-heart and soul-to-soul. It's center-to-center. The way to get to this level of touch is by being relaxed, confident and fully present.

Check in with your receiver to find out what specific types of touch work best for her. For lots of women, what really lights their fire varies from session to session. They often need to do some trial-and-error exploring to find out what the magic move-du-jour is.

Eventually, you'll want to get your other hand involved. Early on, this can be as simple as having four fingers under her buttocks and your thumb resting on her introitus (the opening of her vagina). As she gets more aroused, with permission you'll want to slide a finger or two inside her and start playing with her G-spot. Clitoral stimulation and G-spot play go together wonderfully, kind of like wine and cheese.

Pacing matters a lot in an expanded orgasm session. You want your receiver to linger in her bliss—you want her to relax there and float in her experience. This means backing off sometimes, using a process I call peaking. For instance, you might try stroking her clit eight times, then being still for a count. That will let the arousal settle in and spread. Make a pattern of this: Eight strokes, one pause. Do this for a while, then try variations. Seven strokes and a pause, six strokes and a pause, and so on. Mix newness with repetition—but have that newness be part of a larger pattern. You want to be coherent, not chaotic. Six strokes, pause, six more strokes. Repeat. By peaking her, you maintain and deepen her arousal and avoid sending her out too far too fast, with the inevitable result—she climaxes and crashes, and then it's time to do the dishes.

There's a corollary here: Be patient. The Pointer Sisters like a man with a slow hand. So do I, and so do most women in an expanded orgasm session. I mean three things here. First, make deliberate, controlled motions. Don't speed up because you want more visible results or because you're feeling anxious.

Second, don't jump from one move to another. If something's working, stay with it a while. Repetition can be entrancing—it takes the receiver deeper into her altered state.

Third, don't project impatience. Many guys are often results-oriented. They want to know they're doing a good job, and the feedback they've been conditioned to look for often takes the form of her having screaming orgasms. First of all, women have intense orgasms that take many different forms. Learning to feel energy is your best bet as a giver. Also, men and women have good days and not-so good days. So, men, in your role as giver I encourage you to hold 'doing a good job' differently. Take your time. Be in charge—in a loving, present way. You want to have all your attention on giving her pleasure. She'll love the journey and she'll love you for driving so skillfully. With practice, you'll both get to bask in an ever-increasing variety of amazing orgasmic experiences.

The Big Three

Three principles will get you everything and everywhere in expanded orgasm. Attention, intention and control.

Attention. This is where your mind is focusing at any point in time. In expanded orgasm, you want to have all your attention on your partner when you are the giver. To do this, do your best to stop thinking about yourself. Instead, focus exclusively on your partner. It's not easy, but the good news is that this will become easier as the date progresses and you both slip more deeply into an altered state.

Intention. Prior to the session, you'll have discussed and hopefully agreed upon what you hope to achieve in your expanded orgasm session. Giver, it's your job to hold onto that intention and make sure your goal is achieved. You're the driver. Get her to your shared destination.

Receiver, you also have an intention, but it's not the same one. Your only 'job' is to surrender to pleasure. Your giver is tracking the GPS. Relax and enjoy the ride.

Control. If there's one question that, more than any other, men think but don't ask while they're having sex with someone else, it's probably this: "How am I doing?" It's a competitive world and only natural for men to wonder how they rate.

It's a question born in insecurity—it arises because the guy is worried he may be getting a mediocre or bad grade. Givers, whatever is going on inside your head while you're facilitating an expanded orgasm session, don't let it leak out into the shared space with your partner. Nothing can pop the expanded orgasm balloon faster than anxious, "How am I doing?" energy. Be in charge—in an appropriate and attuned, not controlling, way. You're giving her a gift. Do it with style and grace, not tentatively or apologetically.

I know: This is easier said than done. I'm not minimizing the real challenges givers face. Women are complicated, variable creatures. They're not easy to read, and the clit is a subtle, slippery bit of anatomy—not easy to grasp like your own sturdy cock (assuming that you're a man). No matter. As the giver, your job is to take control. The receiver wants more than anything for you to do this. She desires a strong, confident, knowing, responsive, intent-full, attentive partner to surrender to. Show up as that person.

If this seems like a big hill to climb, I invite you to bear in mind two traps and their simple remedies. First, *silence feeds insecurity.* The more you talk and the more you share—from a place of inquiry and power—the more you'll stay connected with your partner, and the less space those anxious thoughts will have to colonize your mind. Second, *ego feeds insecurity.* The more we think we've got all the answers, the more we believe we know the right way to proceed, the likelier we are to feel embarrassed or worse when things don't go according to plan. Drop the script and the stress drops, too.

During an expanded orgasm session, you are entering a mystery. A double mystery, really—the mystery of the expanded bliss state, and the mystery of the moment. You will show up as powerful and strong to the extent that you also show up as humble, in inquiry, and flexibly able to adapt to what the journey requires. 'Control' isn't a macho concept as I use it here. It's about being strong *and* soft, about knowing where you want to go *and* being flexible in terms of how you get there. Givers, remember this: Confidence isn't synonymous with ego, and power isn't synonymous with inflexibility.

Your partner is saying to you, "I'm turning myself over to you. Hold me and please don't drop me. I'm trusting you to take me for a ride." Giver, accept the challenge and have fun with it. How much can you show your appreciation for her vulnerability and her yearning to trust you? How much can you reward her? How far out can you take her on her ride?

A Short Course for Receivers

A brief anecdote: A few years ago, I went with my partner to a dance class to learn a complicated sequence—it was Zydeco, I believe. For some reason, the teacher started dancing with me. I'm not a particularly good dancer and I didn't know Zydeco. Even so, people kept coming up to us and asking if we were the teachers. The reason: He was a great dancer, and I, thanks to my expanded orgasm practice, was great at surrendering. We worked beautifully together.

There's a moral to this story: Receivers, if you want to have wonderful expanded orgasm sessions, train your giver well. Have them be a wonderful 'dance master.'

That's not all there is to it, of course. You also want to be great at surrendering.

While I encourage you to practice this with a partner, solo-sex sessions are also a great way to develop your capacity to release into pleasure. When you're alone, there's no extra pressure. You can explore and experiment without worrying if you're being a good and desirable partner.

Your orgasms are ultimately your own responsibility. Your partner can facilitate the experience, but they can't cook up orgasms the way they'd prepare you a steak dinner. Even when you have a great partner, when push comes to shove (or tweak comes to stroke), you have to roll your own. So how do you get really good at having orgasms? The same way you get really good at anything else—you practice. Here, too, it's great to do this on your own. Learn your own body. Find out what pleases you. Discover how your body changes, from day to day and from year to year. 'Know thyself,' a sage once said, though I don't think they meant it this way.

Know thyself—and communicate about it, too. Your partner can't always know what you want unless you tell them. This can take the form of words ("A firmer touch, please") or sounds ("Mmm, aaah"). Sounds can be misleading, though. My "this isn't quite working" sound can be the giver's "you're nailing it" sound. If you're going to communicate with sound, make sure you have a shared understanding of what your sounds mean.

I also recommend communicating with yourself. I know this may sound strange. Still, what do you call that move when you circle your clit with medium pressure? Or when you pull apart your labia? If you have a name for it, you can share it with your partner. It creates a sort of shorthand that makes it easier for you to stay out of your head and more in your body when you're having a partnered expanded orgasm session.

You can play 'name that move' with a partner. It's also a fabulous thing to do when pleasuring yourself. It's a great way to get to know what really works for you—and what doesn't.

Here's one more way to take responsibility for your orgasm. Know when something's not working for you—and speak up. It's really disheartening for a giver to be doing their very best to take you out only to discover that they've been taking you in the wrong direction for a while. It creates a lack of trust. If the desire to be nice causes you to be silent, then you're not really being nice at all. You're being cowardly—and unkind. You'll be doing yourself and your giver a service if you notice unpleasurable strokes, or strokes that are not increasing your energy, and make requests for what you do want as soon as possible.

Solo sex is a great way to learn to become more orgasmic. Bear in mind, though, that it's not just about having orgasms. Before any of that, it's about developing the capacity to feel more and to surrender. Build that and you will, um, come.

Talk to Each Other

I've already mentioned this several times, but it's so important I'm giving it a section of its own. Communicating is crucial. Givers, I have three types of sharing in mind:

1. Tell her what you see. "I see a drop of moisture at your introitus." "Your clit just popped out from under the hood." This communicates that you're present and paying attention.
2. Praise your partner. "Your bulbs are puffing up and they look so beautiful." You can't go wrong with this if you're sincere. Many women are plagued by negative thoughts about their genitals. Sincere positive feedback will always be received gratefully.
3. Ask questions. "Is this a good amount of pressure? More? Less?" Keep the questions simple, requiring only a yes or a no reply, so your receiver doesn't have to do a lot of mental processing and can stay in her trance while responding.

Receivers, you have a responsibility here, too. Let your partner know what's working and how to make it better (if you know). This can be tricky—givers can be sensitive to criticism. I recommend starting off with a positive before getting to the request. "I love that you're going really slowly. Now go a little slower, please?" Theoretically, the initial positive feedback will be enough to keep the giver from slipping into an "I'm doing it wrong" mindset. As a practical matter, though, the first words of praise often end up getting discounted or ignored. One partner told me, "As soon as I hear you going into what I think will be the feedback formula, I zone out and wait to be told what I need to be doing differently." So now I often simply ask for what I want. I'll say, for example, "Go a little slower, please." And then (upon the request being done) I'll say, "Thanks, babe!"

The best advice I can give on this subject is that you consult with your partner about what works for them. If they want a 'positivity package,' give it to them. If they don't, that's fine too. Don't be guided by hard-and-fast rules. Do what works best for the two of you.

Being in the giver's role can be challenging—after all, it's hard to maintain complete attention. It's easy to start thinking about the bills that need paying, the ache in your knee, your apparent inability to ever 'do it right,' or how frustrating women are with their endless variability! The list is endless.

Stroke Quality—Playing Her Instrument Elegantly

Givers, here are some things to look out for when you're pleasuring your partner.

Angle of Finger. Notice how your finger makes contact with your partner's clitoris. Ideally, your palm will be resting on her pubic mound with a sense of firmness. Experiment with varying the angle of your finger from almost perpendicular (straight up) to nearly flat. Most women prefer a nearly flat finger.

One Finger Versus Several Fingers. Experiment with using one finger, then mix in the use of two or even three fingers.

Friction Versus Through the Skin. With friction, the surface area is stimulated. With through-the-skin motions, the area below the surface is stimulated in the absence of friction. Because people have changing preferences from moment to moment, there's no 'right way' to do this. Communicate!

Dragging Along. You can go smoothly over the surface, or you can drag your fingers so as to create a sort of wave under the skin. You can learn to do these moves by practicing on yourself.

Evenness of the Experience. Be consistent! Stroke as evenly as possible. Ideally, your stroke will be as smooth as silk.

Feel What She's Feeling. Get out of your head and into hers. And into her physical experience, too. Try to experience what you're doing from, so to speak, her side of the bed.

Make Sure Every Stroke Feels Great to You. If what you're doing doesn't feel wonderful to you, it probably won't feel wonderful to her, either. The more you can be in your pleasure, the more she'll be pleased, too.

Listen To Your Intuition. If your inner voice tells you something, pay attention. If your fingers tell you something, pay even more attention. Ultimately, this is how you'll know what to do next—and the odds that you'll get it right increase in direct proportion to the extent to which you've absorbed basic principles of expanded-orgasm pleasuring like repetition, peaking and going slow.

(Receiver, if he goes with his intuition and gets it wrong, let him know—kindly and considerately.)

Adapted from Expanded Orgasm: Soar to Ecstasy at Your Lover's Every Touch, Second Edition, by Patricia Taylor, Ph.D. (Sourcebooks, 2014)

Receivers, if your giver has moments of distraction—or minutes of distraction, for that matter—have compassion. Bring them back gently to the here-and-now. It's really difficult to be present and even more challenging to stay that way. A kind few words ("You're doing great!")—or even a sweet "yum"—can be all that's needed to bring the giver back into a positive space.

Love, caring and tenderness need to go both ways in an expanded orgasm session.

When Obstacles Arise

Expanded orgasm doesn't always go as planned. You'll have good days and bad days. There'll also be times inside a generally great experience where the ride gets a little bumpy. Don't be surprised when this happens. Expect it. It's part of the journey.

This advice is for both givers and receivers: If things get really out of focus, communicate with your partner that you want to take a break from the action, then stop what you're doing. Take a moment to breathe and get centered. Step away from your hyper-active brain. Put a little smile on your lips—attitude is everything!—and start again.

Distracting thoughts can be annoyingly persistent, though. This basic 'get it together' counsel may not be enough. If you continue to have trouble being present, try this exercise. Visualize a red dot. See it very clearly. Then imagine taking all those intrusive thoughts and packing them inside the dot. You're no longer the 'owner' of the thoughts. The red dot is. So now you can talk to it. "Red dot, you can do what you want with these distractions. You can leave my body and go far away with them, or you can dissolve inside my body so they're no longer trapped in my head. Red dot, it's up to you now. Take them away."

If you're going to take more than a few moments to do this, it's best to take a break from your expanded orgasm session. It'll take you too far away from the mood and sensations of the moment. I recommend this if your challenges are making you feel really stuck: Agree to a break, do the red dot exercise, then come back to having fun.

You can also do a short-form version of the exercise. Simply see your messy thoughts, bundle them into the red dot, and let the dot either integrate with the rest of you, or vanish 'off site.' The short form exercise can be done in seconds—and thus inside a date—without taking focus away from the experience you are sharing or requiring a break. People usually have more success with the short form if they've familiarized themselves with the process first.

In the abstract, this may sound silly. In my experience, it's effective, though—and you can always customize it to make it work better for you. Don't like the red dot? Try a cloud of energy-droplets seeking to dissolve. Will they immerse into nothingness inside you—or float away? Use whatever works best for you.

There's a larger point here. Expanded orgasm isn't only an amazing journey into pleasure. It's also a spiritual practice in the same sense that meditation, yoga and tai chi are spiritual practices. During expanded orgasm sessions, both the giver and receiver learn to be more present and more focused. We learn to be kinder and more compassionate, both to ourselves and to our partner. As the receiver, we learn to go into the Bliss that awaits us beyond our egos—the same Bliss I discovered during my near-death experience.

In short, expanded orgasm is a wonderful way to become a better and happier person.

And to do so while having orgasms. Lots and lots of orgasms.

Now what could be better than that?

SEXY SUMMARY

EXPANDED ORGASM IS A PRACTICE. Initially, it is best done independently of your normal bedroom activities. Then it can be integrated into your sensual-sexual life.

EXPANDED ORGASM SESSIONS can be done solo or with a partner.

BENEFITS INCLUDE physical orgasmic bliss, emotional bonding with a partner, intimate mental connection and attention to one another, and profound spiritual experiences.

CLEAR YOUR MIND before starting.

GIVERS, YOU'RE IN CHARGE. Earn her trust. Be present and attentive. Take her out slowly. Follow the moment, not a script.

RECEIVERS, IT'S YOUR JOB to surrender to pleasure. And to feel. Leave everything else to the giver.

COMMUNICATION is a two-way street. Givers, tell your receiver what you see. Compliment her sincerely. Ask for guidance. Receivers, tell your giver what you want. Do so kindly and considerately. Be compassionate.

DON'T EXPECT THINGS always to go perfectly. They won't. Every time they don't, it's an opportunity for you to practice becoming more present, more centered, and to communicate.

EXPANDED ORGASM ISN'T ONLY an amazing erotic experience. It's also a path to becoming a happier, more vibrant person who's brimming with life-force energy.

MICHAEL WINN *has been a seminal teacher of Taoist sexology, medical qigong and inner alchemy meditation in the West for 35 years. He is the founder of Healing Tao University near Asheville, North Carolina. It sponsors the largest program of Taoist Qi skills in the West—20 summer retreats specializing in certification of high level qigong teachers and healers. It has offered the public a wide array of Taoist arts and sciences for 20 years, including Taoist sexual energy cultivation.*

Winn co-wrote Mantak Chia's first seven books, including Bone Marrow Nei Kung, Healing Energy Through the Tao, Chi Nei Tsang: Deep Organ Massage, *and* Awaken Healing Light of the Tao: Microcosmic Orbit. *Winn is author of the much-acclaimed* Way of the Inner Smile: Tao Path to Peace & Self-Acceptance.

What propelled the Healing Tao system to worldwide fame was Winn's co-authoring with Mantak Chia of Taoist Secrets of Love: Cultivating Male Sexual Energy *(1984) and his later editing of* Healing Love: Cultivating Female Sexual Energy. *He practiced Taoist dual cultivation with his lover and wife Joyce Gayheart for 25 years and taught thousands of Westerners the Tao of sexual energy cultivation.*

Winn was two-term president and early founder of the National Qigong Association. After studying with dozens of masters, Winn developed a unique system of personal development that supercharges ordinary qigong with Taoist internal alchemy meditation. The secret 'alchemical agent' that speeds up one's evolution is skill in refining biological sexual energy into a tangible energy body.

Winn has produced 10 home-study courses on Taoist Internal Alchemy for Westerners to explore the spiritual depths of 'whole-body enlightenment,' known in China as immortality. He's led 18 China Dream Trips doing tai chi and qigong in sacred Taoist mountains.

His partner Joyce passed in 2008. Winn lives with his current wife Jem and their infant son Emerald in a log cabin near Asheville, N.C., He plans to build a Chinese temple nearby to host a global center for spiritual science.

For more information: HealingTaoUSA.com.

CHAPTER THIRTEEN

Non-Ejaculatory Male Orgasm

by Michael Winn & Carl Frankel

IN OUR SOCIETY, A MAN'S SEXUAL PROWESS IS OFTEN MEASURED by his ability to get an erection and by how long it takes him, post-ejaculation, to get hard again. If you're a teenager it may just be a matter of minutes before you're ready for the next round, but if you're a senior citizen it can be a day or more. Either way, the basic architecture is the same—you peak, you tumble off the cliff, and it's no more hard wood for a while.

Men understandably interpret this to mean they've got "pause-till-further-notice" stamped on their penis. The entire sex act becomes shaped by this awareness and sex becomes an exercise in ejaculation management. This can be quite a distraction. If you're focused on your fear of not being able to recover an erection, that much less of you is available to open to a loving connection and pleasure.

Many men develop excellent ejaculatory control, but even when it's not an issue, they're still managing their tumble off the cliff. There's another option. You can have all the pleasure of orgasm without ejaculation and its subsequent pause, called the "refractory period" by sexologists. Orgasm and ejaculation are physiologically separate processes. You can have an orgasm and bypass ejaculation entirely by internally recycling your semen.

Using the approach of the ancient Daoist (Taoist) masters, I've been practicing non-ejaculatory orgasm in this manner for more than three decades and I've taught thousands of men how to do this. It's quite simple if you're willing to open your mind to the Daoist energetic perspective on how the body operates.

When you cultivate non-ejaculatory orgasm, you get that looming refractory period out of your head and your sex life. You can enjoy the male equivalent of female extended orgasms, with the pleasure lasting minutes, even hours and days. This is full-on, whole-body orgasmic pleasure, not some pale shadow. Bypassing the emission of semen doesn't remove the deepest pleasure of orgasm.

For the man who's mastered non-ejaculatory orgasm, there's no more worry about a post-squirting collapse. You are completely free to play energetically with your lover and are able to sustain an erection longer because you're not triggering erectile collapse with a full ejaculation.

The Physiology of Orgasm

Sperm are stored in the epididymis, which is located in the testicles. At any given moment, hundreds of millions of those little fellas live there, ready to emerge in a single ejaculation. When they're in a passive, unaroused state, they just relax and float around like they're in a spa. It's warm and liquid in there—things are, like, mellow, dude! When you see a sexy person or start having a sexual fantasy, suddenly that laid-back spa turns into a disco. All those sperm start dancing around in a frenzy and it gets really crowded and hot. If it turns into full-on sex, before long the sperm are going, "There isn't room for all 500 million of us in this disco."

Inevitably, the energy reaches a bursting point and those sperm head for the exit. In your standard ejaculatory orgasm, they're shot up a tube called the vas deferens to the prostate, which adds a clear liquid called prostatic fluid to the sperm. This liquid, also known as pre-cum, contains nutrients that give them strength and energy as they head off on their epic longshot journey through the urethra, out the penis and up the vaginal canal through the uterus and into the Fallopian tubes to the Promised Land of Egg.*

It's as if the prostate is handing them a little lunchbox. *Thanks, Mom!* And off they go on their way.

The first part of the male ejaculatory process is testicular. It sends sperm up the vas deferens. The second is prostatic and it sends those little swimmers out the penis. When you practice non-ejaculatory orgasm, you allow the testicular pulsation to happen, but not the prostatic pulsation. You re-route the sexual energy so it moves up and inside your body instead of out the penis.

The physical sperm, once emptied of their essence (called *jing qi* by Daoists), are absorbed back into the bloodstream from the testicles, vas deferens, prostate and bladder. Their valuable minerals and proteins are recycled and put to good use by the blood.

*** Evolution doesn't know about blow jobs.**

Health and Non-Ejaculatory Orgasm

If you're choosing to orgasm without ejaculating, it's very important for health reasons to move the energy up inside the body rather than leave it to stagnate in the genito-urinary tract. I've seen research studies which suggest that men who practice conventional celibacy have a higher rate of prostate cancer than other men. While the findings are far from conclusive, if true, this is probably because their sexual energy gets trapped in their prostate. According to Chinese medicine, stagnant energy is what creates tumors. If they were practicing non-ejaculatory orgasm, they'd be moving the energy, it wouldn't be stagnant and their rates of prostate cancer would likely decline.

One Daoist practice for keeping men from ejaculating is to have them or their partner press firmly on the Million Dollar Spot, located on the man's perineum. When you press this, you're compressing the vas deferens. It's an effective way to keep sperm from moving into the prostate and losing your *jing qi*.

But after years of working with Daoist sexology, this is one of their few practices I've disavowed because it creates congestion. You're trapping those 500 million disco dancers in the testicles, which may cause 'blue balls,' and that's not healthy. You want that energy to move. You don't want it dammed up.

We all know how powerful sexual energy is. When you circulate it through your body instead of sending it out your penis, it's like you're super-charging yourself with a dose of the best nutrients ever. I'm in my mid-sixties and have been practicing non-ejaculatory orgasm for well over three decades. During that time, I've had only a few ejaculatory orgasms. I have no gray hair and people tell me I have the energy of a man in my forties. While this is only my subjective experience, I attribute this largely to conservation of my sexual seed. I've had amazing sex and I recently made a baby with my new wife, who's in her twenties. We waited till her fertile time, I elected to have an ejaculatory orgasm, and we succeeded on our first try.

I believe this method of internally recycling sexual energy supercharges your sperm when you do finally release it, producing extraordinarily healthy children. While one case isn't scientific proof, in a world where so many people face fertility challenges and where guys in their 60s tend to have less peppy sperm than younger men, I am living testimony to the health and vitality benefits of practicing non-ejaculatory orgasm. It certainly doesn't inhibit fertility, and I've been enjoying high-energy 'spiritual' orgasms for decades!

Let me emphasize that I made a strong commitment to 100% non-ejaculatory orgasm. Practice makes perfect. Nothing requires you to do the same. How much you practice non-ejaculatory orgasm is entirely up to you. You can do it as much or as little as you like. Even doing it half the time you make love or masturbate will provide major health and spiritual benefits.

If you want to practice non-ejaculatory orgasm, you'll need to put effort into developing the ability. It's not difficult to learn, but you can't get it by snapping your fingers, either. How long it takes to master non-ejaculatory orgasm varies from person to person. Factors include the emotional and physical blocks you're carrying in your body and how long they've been there, and your comfort level with the Daoist energy model. Some men pick it up quickly, others more slowly—but I know from long experience that any man can learn it.

It's About Energy . . .

As a boy and young man, I had way more sexual energy than I knew what to do with. I had endless crushes on girls and masturbated three times a day. Eventually I realized that all my obsessing about sex wasn't enhancing my life. I wanted to control this incredibly strong urge instead of having it control me and so I started exploring various spiritual practices, including kundalini yoga.

Eventually my path brought me to a Daoist, Mantak Chia. As a young man, he had been told that his sexual energy was exhausted and he would die if he didn't do something about it. He learned non-ejaculatory orgasm as a way to heal himself. Thus, we had different but parallel paths. His sexual energy was depleted and mine was excessive, but we both had a sexual energy problem, and we both healed ourselves by practicing non-ejaculatory orgasm.

We were men on a non-emission.

Mantak Chia's English wasn't good. I ended up writing his first seven books. *Taoist Secrets of Love: Cultivating Male Sexual Energy* sold hundreds of thousands of copies and propelled him to fame.

I've evolved my teaching of non-ejaculatory orgasm beyond what Mantak taught me, as I found Westerners need to do important emotional clearing work to be truly successful in the practice. My preferred methods involve the Six Healing Sounds and emotional alchemy, known to Daoists as Fusion of the Five Elements. The Healing Sounds use acupuncture channels with sound and arm movements to release trapped emotional energy in our vital organs that can block the flow of sexual energy. (I discuss Fusion of the Five Elements below.)

When we practice non-ejaculatory orgasm, we're practicing energy management. Not energy as in petroleum or electricity, but energy as in the mysterious, ineffable force that underlies everything and moves through us all.

The Chinese focus on energy first and matter second. The Chinese word for energy is *chi* (also spelled *qi*, both pronounced *chee*). This *chi* flow, or life force, is the root of what make us feel alive. It's totally embedded in the Chinese language. A friend of mine counted 647 words in his Chinese dictionary that integrate the character for *chi*. The word for garlic translates as 'hot *chi*.' The word for weather is 'atmospheric *chi*.'

In Western culture, we pay much less attention to energy. We're more focused on the level that vibrates more slowly—the physical body. But it's energy that creates the body, and it's energy that makes a body feel well or ill, sexy or ugly and unloved.

In the Daoist view, there's nothing esoteric or mystical about chi. It's understood for what it is, as what precedes and underlies all manifestations into form. Everything that exists, from rocks to people to planets, is vibrating with energy.

There's *chi* in our thoughts, feelings and perceptions as well as in our physical selves. Someone insults us and we feel angry. Anger has its own unique quality of energy—we all know what it feels like. When we do a practice like qigong or tai chi, we're working with the energy that underlies those thoughts, feelings and perceptions. We're creating the possibility of rewriting our habitual scripts. We're tinkering with our energetic DNA. Daoist methods of energy management can help us transmute this anger into compassion and love.

. . . And It's About Sex

For Daoists, everything is sexual. I don't mean this in the Western sense of being randy. The Daoist view of sex is premised in observation, not arousal. They observe nature and see a profoundly sexual process, with the entire universe emerging out of a marriage between the male principle, yang, and the female principle, yin.

The Daoist view is that *the entire universe is in a constant state of sexual procreation*. Behind the world of visible form, there is a formless world. Formless energies are polarized into male (yang) and female (yin) aspects, and it is their sexual commingling that creates the world of form. Light and shadow, solar and lunar, penetrating and receptive—these are some of the polarities that shape the world.

Imagine a baby before it's born. It's pure potential; it doesn't exist yet. It takes a male sperm and a female egg to turn that potential into something physical. Everything in the universe is created the same way. Masculine and feminine transform the formless into form.

Our cells are always reproducing themselves—this is sexual. Our yin and yang aspects are constantly interacting on physical-sexual, emotional, mental, and spiritual levels. And just like the cosmos itself, we humans are constantly performing the sexual act of transmuting spirit into body, the formless into form.

In the Daoist view, we have an energy portal where this happens. Think of it as a Star Trek portal with a vapor lock in the middle. One door—the *mingmen*, or 'gate of destiny'—is located between the two kidneys, at the level of our navel. The *chi* in the mingmen is formless, waiting to be born as both our body and our destiny. The other door is the *dantian* ("elixir field"). It's located in the exact same space as the mingmen, only it holds the slower vibration of our physical essence.

The formless spiritual *chi* comes into the *mingmen*, where it becomes sexually polarized into the two forces of yin and yang. It then passes into the *dantian* and from there it creates your body through a network of acupuncture meridians. This is the energy that fuels you as you go through your life. It's also the energy we work with when practicing non-ejaculatory orgasm.

All creation is sexual, and that sexual polarity is what connects us to everyone and everything.

The Weirdness Factor

When the subject of Chinese energy healing is raised, some people get dismissive. They see it as mystical, pseudo-scientific and a sad excuse for medicine, on a par with medieval leeching. This attitude is totally misguided and unscientific. On my website, I've posted a summary of 3,500 studies supporting the efficacy of medical qigong and energy healing. Harvard recently came out with a book on using tai chi to heal all kinds of chronic illness. Collectively the evidence establishes beyond a doubt that Chinese energy healing works.

> ***The secret to long life and spiritual orgasm is to internally capture and transmute our sexual energy rather than ejaculating it out of our body.***

The Chinese and specifically Daoist body-centered approach to energy flow is actually more accessible for Westerners than most other-dimensional Eastern spiritual traditions. Take Zen, which is about completely stilling your mind. This usually translates into repressing one's sexual vibration in order to return to the formless chi state. Trying to do this is very difficult, if not impossible, for most Westerners. Is it even desirable?

Daoist internal alchemy, by contrast, is about practicing internal sex. Since everyone knows how sex works, they're being asked to do something that's much more intuitively accessible than 'stilling the mind.' The Daoist starting point is, "How do I have sex inside myself?" The answer: We build up our reservoirs of masculine and feminine energy and then sexually couple them. This produces an internal orgasm that overflows partly into the physical body and partly into our original spiritual state of formless *chi*. This is much better suited for the Western mind than other forms of meditation because there are dynamic actions to be taken here.

Practicing non-ejaculatory orgasm is entirely natural and healthy. It's not Daoism that's weird, it's Western culture that's weird with its excessive yang emphasis on external achievement and doing, doing, doing. Sexually, this shows up as an excess of ejaculation. In Eastern cultures, there's a healthier balance between yang projection on the one hand and yin receptivity and surrender on the other. There's a greater tendency to look inward: "What's going on inside me?" When we do this, notions like internal sexual alchemy start seeming totally normal and not weird.

A Short How-To

You're probably familiar with acupuncture, which uses needles to affect energy flows. It's an effective technique, but it has its limits because needles can only go so deep. Below the twelve vital organ meridians that can be accessed via acupuncture, there are eight deeper meridians. In Daoist medicine, they're called the Eight Extraordinary Vessels. I think of them as the channels of your soul.

Two of these eight meridians flow around our torso via the back (spine) and front (chest). When the two deep channels flow as one, this is called by Daoists the Microcosmic Orbit. The Governing Vessel, or fire channel, is yang. It runs from the perineum up the spine to the top of the head and down to the mouth. The Conception Vessel, or water channel, is yin. It runs from the perineum up the front of the body to the mouth. When we energetically mix the spine's fire yang (masculine *chi*) and the front water yin (feminine *chi*), we are alchemically mixing sexual forces inside our body and regulating, by extension, the balance of yin-yang *chi* flowing through the other six deep and 12 superficial organ meridians.

When we work with these eight deep meridians, there's a spillover effect—the 12 shallower meridians are affected. It's as if you're improving the flow in your plumbing, only it's energy, not water, that's running through the pipes. One of the pipes has hot water and the other has cold water. You connect them and get a balanced water flow. This is healthy ... and it feels great, too.

When you circulate orgasmic *chi* around the body rather than out the penis, it is easiest to first work with the Governing and Conception Vessels.

You're basically being a traffic cop and sending the energy up one channel and down the other. It's a straightforward mechanical operation. You don't have to be a high-level meditator to do this. You just need a good map of how your body and sexual energy flow really work.

The best way to make this happen is with a combination of breathing, visualizing and your ability to feel sexual energy. There's a strong connection between intention, visualization, breath, and physical effects. Western science hasn't explained it yet, but it's real.

When we imagine energy moving, we're essentially giving the process permission to unfold. We're giving it our blessing; we're putting aside our distractions and skepticism and being a cheerleader. If a child is learning to ride a bicycle, it will probably figure it out one way or the other. If Mom and Dad are there cheering it on, it'll probably learn faster. That's what conscious, active breath and visualization do. They create a space for positive results to happen.

Chi flows where the mind goes, the Daoists say.

So now you're having sex. Maybe with yourself, maybe with someone else. And you've decided to practice non-ejaculatory orgasm. What exactly do you do?

Start early. Once those disco dancers are all heated up and about to head out the door, it may be too late to stop them from shooting out the penis.

Starting very early in arousal, do what's called the 'cool draw' or 'testicle breathing.' It starts with becoming aware of your testicles. You may want to put a hand on them and feel their warmth. Focus your attention, breathe into them gently and eventually you'll feel a little tingle. Then turn your lips into a smile and start breathing that energy up your body.

You have three options here. You can breathe the energy up your spine (Governing Vessel), up the front of your body (Conception Vessel), or directly into your *dantian* (*belly center*), where *chi* will build up until it spontaneously overflows up the core channel in the center of the body. Whichever path you select, imagine you've got a straw inside your body and are sucking the energy upward from your testicles.*

Locate this imaginary straw in the area of your testicles and use the path that works best for you. For most men, the back spine channel is more open than their front channel, so that's often easier to work with.

Whichever channel you use, eventually you'll feel the energy in your head. If you pull the sexual energy into your dantian, it may flow straight up the core channel through your heart and eventually to the head. Once *chi* flows to the head from the front or back channel, let it flow down the opposite

---

*** Women can do a similar exercise focusing on their ovaries.**

channel. If it comes up the central channel, it can flow down both spine and chest, or just the one that is most open. When you do this, you're cycling your sexual energy. Your male energy is firing up your female energy and your female energy is powering up your male energy in an ongoing, mutually reinforcing 'virtuous cycle.'

This is the sexual version of the Microcosmic Orbit. It's called this because it's a miniature version of what unfolds at the macro-cosmic level, where yin mixes with yang in the ongoing sexual process of creation that births stars, planets, and all creatures.

I recommend first learning cool draw testicle breathing when you're neither aroused nor having sex. You're developing an energetic pathway. The more you use it, the more clear and unobstructed it becomes. It's much easier to clear the brush away without the distractions of arousal and partner play.

I also encourage my students, especially beginning ones, to support the process by squeezing, or clenching and unclenching, their muscles. When you do this, you pull blood to the area you're working. *Chi flows where the blood goes*, the Daoists also say. When you get an erection, your penis engorges with blood—that's why you have so much energy there. If you want to move sexual energy away from your penis, you'll want to move the blood elsewhere. You do this by working other muscles.

Begin by clenching the muscles in the area of your perineum until the urge to ejaculate subsides. This slows the sexual charge of sperm flowing to your penis. Then squeeze and pulse the *gluteus maximus*—your buttocks. This is the largest muscle in your body and it draws a huge amount of blood to it. When the blood goes there, the sexual energy is drawn with it. You're moving it away from the path of unconscious ejaculation out the penis.

Sexual chi flows where your mind goes.

You can also tighten the muscles around the spine and your neck muscles. You can even tighten your fists. There's no right way here—find out what works best for you, remembering that your larger goal is to redirect your blood flow so it's less concentrated in your penis and spread more throughout your body. This is a quick way to divert sexual energy away from imminent ejaculation out the penis.

A key to doing non-ejaculatory orgasm effectively is to be relaxed. But how can you relax if you're doing all this muscle-clenching? There are two answers. The first is that muscle-clenching is optional. It's a good way to learn to move sexual energy in the beginning, but once you've got your energy pathways open, especially by mastering Testicle Breathing, you won't need to clench any more. Second, there are levels of relaxation. You can be tensing your muscles at one level and relaxed at another, higher energetic level. Put a smile on your face and have fun!

Challenges and Obstacles

Over the years, I've found that some women don't want their man to practice non-ejaculatory orgasm. Often it's because they feel as if they are losing a gift from their lover. Their man may be emotionally aloof and not give much of himself. His seed is a stand-in for his love and they don't want to give that up.

Even ungiving men usually want to make their woman sexually happy. If this means ejaculating, well, then they'll ejaculate. It's the least they can do—in the positive and negative senses of the term.

An entirely different story about ejaculation is out there waiting to be embraced. When men practice non-ejaculatory orgasm, they're recycling sexual energy into their heart, lips and hands where they can share it with their partner. They're still giving their woman the gift of their sexuality, but it's more fully embodied and more powerful.

When women partners come to understand the bigger gift they're getting, they often let go of their attachment to male ejaculation. They know that they're really getting their man this time, in a more full and connected way. They are getting his whole (sexualized) body and soul love.

I've also known many male gay couples that dramatically improved their relationship using these techniques. They'd been stuck in a pattern of male-to-male quickie 'rabbit sex' and it wasn't very satisfying for either of them. Then one or both started practicing non-ejaculatory orgasm and this led to deeper, more profound exchanges with their partner.

It's not only partners who get attached to ejaculation. The seed owners themselves do, too. This male attachment is emotional, not erotic. It's how they've always had sex and they've come to see it as the act's ultimate gratification and reward.

Sexual energy is very bonding. That's one reason breaking up is so difficult. In your rational mind, you may know you're not right for each other, but sex creates powerful attachments and it can be very difficult to let go. We also bond to our fantasies. If you get off on the idea of being catered to sexually by many eager playmates, you'll get attached to that notion. When we have a hot fantasy, we're super-gluing our psyche to that turn-on.

While there's nothing inherently wrong with this, it can be a problem with regard to non-ejaculatory orgasm. You're not practicing internal sexual alchemy when you project your erotic energy onto one of these fantasies. This is why I advise men to put one hand on their heart when they masturbate. This shifts the energy flow from the typical male path of genitals to spine to head, which bypasses the heart. Putting your hand on your heart and sending sexual love to your soul deep within triggers a process of heart-centered sexual alchemy. You're mixing heart energy with sex energy and bringing the whole body into the mix.

If you have (or need) a special sexual fantasy to get turned on, use it to get aroused, but then direct it to either a real current lover or to your own heart. This keeps you from projecting all that sexual chi onto the object of your fantasy, which has the undesirable result of dissipating the energy rather than having it nourish your body.

Sex is a magnet that attracts and then holds many energetic and emotional blockages in our subconscious. If we want our energetic pipes to flow freely, we need to clean out the muck that attaches to our sexuality. I recommend a mix of practices for this.

The first is the Inner Smile meditation, which is the easiest meditation ever. You simply smile throughout your body. You're practicing unconditional acceptance—of yourself, not other people. If stuff comes up, you accept that it exists in your body, smile to it, and let it go. If you can feel it, you can heal it.

I also strongly recommend the ancient Daoist practice of qigong. There are many ways to do this and they're all easy to learn. One qigong practice I teach is called *Five Animals Qigong*. It involves sound, color visualization and arm motion and does a great job of releasing blocked emotional energy.

I also encourage men to practice the Microcosmic Orbit when they're not having sex. When you do this, you're building your capacity to open your front and back channels. Over the years, I've tested many ways to do the Microcosmic Orbit and the one I've found most powerful is the Wudang Spinning Pearl method. Essentially, you create a spinning energy and move it from the sexual center and spin it slowly around the Microcosmic Orbit in your spine and chest. It does a great job of breaking up limiting emotional and mental patterns that have gotten stuck in our bodies. It also makes it much easier to move and ramp up sexual energy throughout the body when the time comes for that.

I strongly recommend that everyone gain skill with this spinning orbit practice *before* attempting to recycle their sexual energy with non-ejaculatory orgasm. It's important to have this pathway open and clear to receive the flow of excited sexual energy. It's best to learn this skill from someone who has experienced it, which is why, in the tradition I was trained in, it is never transmitted in writing, only orally (which fortunately includes audio recordings).

Other Sexual Vitality Qigong movement methods help build up the kidneys and liver, which control much of your sexual robustness.

Serious Business

Practicing non-ejaculatory orgasm isn't something to take lightly. Many people have clogged energetic plumbing due to physical or emotional trauma. If you start moving lots of sexual energy into your upper body before you're physically ready to receive it, the energy can express in unhealthy and uncomfortable ways such as insomnia or the surfacing of unpleasant memories.

You'll have more success practicing non-ejaculatory orgasm if the garden of your body has been readied for all that sexual energy. This is why it's so important to prepare the ground with exercises like the Inner Smile meditation, a movement qigong practice, and the Microcosmic Orbit. Serious students of Daoist sex will also learn emotional alchemy, known as Fusion of the Five Elements. This dissolves negative emotions and old reactive patterns stored in our vital organs that tend to get reinforced by the unconscious flow of sexual energy. Essentially, you 'strip off' the negative charge (e.g., anger) from an emotional pattern and then concentrate the underlying energy into a ball of neutral *chi* formed in the lower dantian (belly). In effect, you recycle and re-digest your unconscious emotional patterns so they actually make you stronger and energetically more clear. Learning Fusion of the Five Elements assures a superior level of success in managing one's emotional and sexual energy as the two transmute into spiritual orgasm.

Practicing non-ejaculatory orgasm is very empowering. *Literally.* It opens your *dantian* so you can take in more *chi* from both the inner planes and the outer world—it fires you up energetically. Make sure you can handle the increase in personal power you'll get from doing these energetic self-cultivation practices.

In these pages, I've given a short introduction to non-ejaculatory orgasm. Because everyone's sexuality is unique and complex, some may need to customize their practice or seek personal training. This chapter is really just a *taste* of a "how-to." I hope you'll take what I've shared here and use it as the basis of a practice. It's important when you start on this path to *never* feel guilty about ejaculating. Allow your training process to be gradual—some may take years to master non-ejaculatory orgasm, others will get it more quickly. But even partial success can bring you amazing rewards in your sex life and general health as well.

SEXY SUMMARY

Practicing non-ejaculatory orgasm is a natural, healthy activity that can bypass the troublesome refractory period, increase your staying power, and transform your sex life and love relationships for the better.

When you practice non-ejaculatory orgasm, you're performing heart-centered internal sexual alchemy.

Microcosmic Orbit: Work with two deep energy meridians, the yang Governing Vessel and the yin Conception Vessel. They are stabilized by a core central channel and energy centers in your belly, heart, and head.

Testicle breathing: Imagine a straw sucking sexual energy from your testicles into your upper body and ultimately into your head. Then send it back down to your dantian at the navel center.

Clench and unclench your perineum and buttocks to pull sexual energy into your upper body.

Take care to prepare your body to receive all this sexual energy. Recommended practices include the Inner Smile meditation, Sexual Vitality Qigong, Microcosmic Orbit, and emotional alchemy using Fusion of Five Elements.

You are stepping into your power as a male, exercising your right to enjoy a full body orgasm.

Have fun and celebrate your newfound power!

TALLULAH SULIS CHP, CMT, CSB *is a renowned sex educator, Certified Hakomi Therapist, Certified Sexological Bodyworker and Certified Massage Therapist. She is also trained in the Somatica Method.*

*She has travelled around the world teaching workshops and "squirt-shops" to men, women and couples. Tallulah directed and produced a ground-breaking educational film about female ejaculation in 2007—*Divine Nectar: A Guide to Female Ejaculation.

She has been featured in educational videos, radio, books such as The Four Hour Body *by Tim Ferriss, and television shows such as Penn and Teller and Playboy TV. She is an author of several online information products with Personal Life Media.*

As a sex activist, artist and educator, Tallulah is passionate about helping people release shame and feel sexually empowered and radiantly alive. She lives in the Hollywood Hills and sees clients privately for coaching and counseling.

For more information: TherapyInBed.com.

CHAPTER FOURTEEN

Female Ejaculation

by Tallulah Sulis & Carl Frankel

I'M A PROFESSIONAL FEMALE EJACULATION COACH. THAT'S RIGHT: I teach women how to squirt. Can we agree that this is not your usual profession? It's certainly not a career I planned on while growing up!

If female ejaculation were simply a technical skill—a parlor trick—I wouldn't be devoting my life to it. But it's much more than that. The journey it sends you on can be ecstatic, empowering, emotional and cathartic all at once. It can take you into the depths of your being. It can also be quite profound to share this level of intimacy and vulnerability with your partner.

I teach female ejaculation because it's spiritually and emotionally transformative. It's a path and it's a revelation.

Best of all, this mind-blowing and ecstatic experience is totally learnable. Just about every woman can develop the capacity to gush. In fact, you may already have ejaculated without knowing it!

Tallulah Learns to Squirt

I didn't gush—at least, not consciously—until I was in my early 20s. I had recently graduated from Sarah Lawrence College, which has a sexually liberated culture, and I felt quite knowledgeable about sex. I had a wonderful lover who at some point said, "I think you can ejaculate." I couldn't really relate to it. For me, it was like a circus act or something you'd see in a sex show, along the lines of women shooting ping-pong balls out of their vaginas. But the next time we were having sex, for some reason, I let go in a slightly deeper way when I came, and my partner said, "There, you just squirted."

My response was, "I did?" I had a vague sense that something different had happened, but it was subtle, not explosive or dramatic. The bed wasn't soaked. I wasn't even aware that I had gushed.

It was a mind-blowing experience anyway. It wasn't the physical ejaculation that triggered my sense of exhilarating overwhelm so much as the permission my unconscious had given me to let go just that little bit more. This very slight shift felt like much more than that to me. It was as if something epic and magnificent had just occurred that had implications not only for me, but for all humanity. All sorts of questions started to come up for me. Why didn't more women know about this? Why had I assumed this wasn't possible or some sort of parlor trick? Why was so little information available about ejaculation and the process of letting go that seemed to be part of it? Why did this feel so important to me?

I'll admit it: I became a bit obsessive. Over time I became like a mad scientist, practicing on my own and with my partner as well. It was a very personal and empowering journey for me. I didn't want to have to rely on someone else to provide the experience; I wanted to own it for myself. And so I embarked upon a journey of discovery. I became an 'ejacu-naut.'

The more I explored, the more I learned, and the more I learned, the more adept I became at ejaculating. My G-spot became more responsive and sensitive and I grew increasingly skilled at surrendering more deeply. Going into my ejaculatory space became almost like a game for me. How fully could I experience my pleasure? How deeply could I go into the realm of unbounded permission and surrender?

Progress was made. Much progress. Over time, what had started out as a tiny squirt evolved into a capacity to have ejaculatory experiences that took me incredibly far out emotionally, spiritually and erotically....and drenched me, my lover and the entire bed!

I had empowered myself to surrender profoundly and I felt like a superstar squirt-goddess!

It has been a wet and wild ride of tapping into a sacred and profound experience I had never known was even possible. I love teaching about female ejaculation because it is such an honor to help women open up and tap into their amazing sexual potential.

The Impact of Pornography

Culturally there's a lot of confusion about female ejaculation. If you go to the Wikipedia entry on the G-spot, you will find this claim: "Neither the G-spot nor the existence of female ejaculation has been proven." I understand the confusion about the G-spot because it's misnamed and misunderstood. But dubiousness about the existence of female ejaculation despite all the squirting you see in porn and the massive anecdotal evidence of everyone who's done or witnessed it? In the name of science, these skeptics are being silly. Both female ejaculation and the G-spot do exist.

That's not our only confusion about gushing. For many of our other misunderstandings, we have porn to thank:

- It presents squirting as a one-dimensional technical feat, sort of like the parlor trick I referred to earlier.
- It depicts female ejaculation as something that is forced out aggressively with little to no warm-up. While female ejaculation can be expelled by pushing out, it can also be released more gently. It also is more apt to happen once a woman has had ample warm-up time and stimulation to her G-spot. She often needs to be in a highly aroused state, and getting there can take time—much more time than is usually depicted in wham-bam porn displays.
- It cheapens a beautiful and profound experience. In porn, female ejaculation is often presented as a sort of competitive sport. *How far can you squirt? I can squirt farther!* Female ejaculation as a lewd variation on a watermelon seed-spitting contest is a long, long way from the multidimensional experience it can be.

Pornography also creates a sense of obligation for many women. They see women on the Internet squirt and decide that unless they deliver those same gushing goods, their partners will view them as inadequate. This pressure, plus how it's depicted in porn, can cause some women to feel disdain and even repulsion for female ejaculation.

To be sure, pornography's influence isn't all bad. Lots of women learn about female ejaculation from watching X-rated material. To the extent that porn educates women about their sexual potential, it's made a positive contribution. But its porn depiction has downsides, too.

The Physiology of Female Ejaculation

What actually happens when a woman squirts?

If you put your fingers into a vagina and turn them upward, they will make contact with a ribbed, cylindrical mound of tissue that extends two or three inches into the opening along the roof of the vagina, almost as far as the cervix. When you do this, you're making indirect contact with the urethral sponge, which wraps around the entire urethra.

Although not mentioned much, the urethral sponge is an essential piece of female sexual equipment. It's full of erectile tissue, the same material that causes penises to swell and grow hard.

If you stroke the urethral sponge crosswise, window wiper-style, or lengthwise with a 'come hither' motion, it will become engorged and swell up. This is a delightful experience for the owner of said vagina—but only if she's at high-level arousal (which isn't always the case).

You probably know the urethral sponge by another name. Yes, folks, this is the G-spot, the very same piece of female genital anatomy whose existence Wikipedia tells us is suspect. To be fair, one can understand the confusion. If women, their partners, and genital scientists go into the vagina looking for a hyper-sensitive 'spot,' they won't find it. Because it's not there. What they will find is a length of tissue that gets swollen and juicy when stimulated. One or more parts of the sponge may be especially sensitive in some women, which is why the erectile sponge can be experienced as a super-juicy spot. The area behind the spongy mound where it starts to narrow is often the most highly sensitive spot for women. Another common hot spot is at the front of the urethral sponge right near the vaginal opening. But it's the entire sponge that gets puffy.

The urethral sponge contains a network of glandular tubules called the Skene's (or paraurethral) glands. They are enmeshed in the sponge's erectile tissue and have about 30 openings along the length of the urethra as well as two main ducts that open just inside or outside the urethral orifice.

While there's no scientific consensus on the matter, sex teacher, medical professional and fellow contributor Sheri Winston makes a compelling case that these glands are the source of female ejaculate. She also postulates that the main source of all that liquid is the bloodstream (blood is mostly water). The water from the blood diffuses through the capillary wall and enters the glandular tubule. There it mixes with the products of the glandular cells and becomes the elixir we call female ejaculate. From the tubules the fluid empties via the ducts into the urethra. From there, it's either expelled out the opening or it backs up into the bladder and comes out with the next urination.

Squirting is a journey, not a competitive sport or destination.

Winston believes that female ejaculate has immunological properties. The orifices of the body are inviting ports of call for organisms that cause infection. The urethra is a particularly risky opening because it's near both the anus and the vagina. The microbes that live inside the anus belong there but not elsewhere, and the vagina tends to attract disease-bearing visitors like hands, mouths and penises. The bacteria they carry can cause urinary tract and other infections. Vulnerable openings such as the urethra and vagina need guards at the gate. If Winston is correct, the ejaculate cleanses the urethral opening of these harmful bacteria.

Thousands of years ago, female ejaculate was revered for its health benefits. Practitioners of Ayurveda (the traditional medicine of India) and Tantra called it amrita, Sanskrit for the nectar of life. Taoist sexuality students and practitioners of traditional Chinese healing called it white moon flower medicine. These folks were probably onto something.

The Varieties of Female Ejaculation

Gushing can take you on many different journeys. Sometimes it's very yin (this is the Taoist term for soft and surrendering; it's typically associated with the feminine) and at other times it's yang (more masculine, more forceful and directed). There are times when my body feels like it's melting, letting go—this is yin. On some occasions, my response is more yang and emphatic: I want to celebrate like a football player who just scored a touchdown. There are times when my pleasure is in the tangibility of the experience. I can also experience a positive association with child-bearing. I call it "giving birth to your orgasm" when you bear down with your pelvic floor muscles to both push out and release the ejaculate. This feels wonderful and aah, what a release!

There are times when I gush explosively. *Look, a geyser!*

Sometimes it's as if a dam breaks. The ejaculate flows and flows, but I'm flooding, not squirting.

Sometimes I produce just a few drops when I ejaculate.

On porn, you often see women squirting in a grand arc, as if they were fountains. Don't expect this to happen or assume you're not 'doing it right' if you don't. Whether or not you produce a fountain when you gush depends on many factors, including your physical position, exactly where your urethra is located and where it's pointing, where you are in your menstrual cycle and how strong your pelvic floor muscles are.

Don't get caught up in trying to 'do it right' or 'do it more.' Squirting is a journey, not a competitive sport or destination.

There's no predicting exactly what type of ejaculation you'll have and there's no sure way to make yourself have one type of ejaculation and not another. Which is fine, because all squirts, gushes, geysers and droplets are created equal.

And then there's female ejaculation's relationship to orgasm. If we define female orgasm as a series of measurable clitoral and/or vaginal contractions, it's a simple matter to address. Ejaculation can happen just prior to, during or independently of a woman's genital orgasm. But let's think bigger here.

People can have whole-body orgasms that aren't genitally centered. These are real orgasms even though they don't fit the narrow technical definition. If we understand orgasm in its more inclusive sense as an escalating ecstatic state that may or may not include localized genital contractions, then ejaculation is orgasmic in and of itself.

Learning to Ejaculate

Not every woman who wants to ejaculate needs to learn how to do so. Squirting comes naturally for some women. I've read that 6-8% of women are natural ejaculators. That number strikes me as about right.*

If you're not in this small minority and want to learn to squirt, this section is for you.

How difficult is it to learn? That depends on the woman. Some pick it up right away, for others it's a matter of time and practice, and for a small minority of women, the challenges are so great they never get there. Many women find it useful to witness a demo. This gives them a visceral understanding of the experience that they can't get from talking or reading.

I've taught classes where one-quarter of the women in attendance gushed during the workshop. Considering the relatively public nature of these sessions, that's an impressive number. Many others learn to ejaculate during their private practice sessions after they've been to a workshop or seen my DVD.

It's not uncommon to encounter challenges or blocks while learning to gush. The main reason women don't ejaculate is because they don't know it exists, so it never occurs to them to learn how to do it. Shame, emotional blocks, not knowing one's body well enough, fear of making a mess, problems surrendering, misinformation and the absence of high arousal are other reasons women have trouble ejaculating. The good news is that all these issues can be overcome.

In order to ejaculate, two distinct types of know-how are required. The first is emotional and the second is physical. Let's start with the emotional piece, which is where women often face the deepest challenges. As I've indicated, a key to ejaculating is surrendering to the process—letting it unfold. While to some extent letting go comes naturally, it's also something we need to learn. In order to surrender more deeply, we need to *intend* to surrender more deeply. Ironically this mental set, this *intending*, can interfere with the actual surrendering. When we intend, it's easy to get into a yang frame of mind:

*** I've also read that 55-60% of women have ejaculated at least once in their life. This number seems wildly inflated, but only if you exclude all the women who've have had mini-ejaculations without knowing it. Put these 'innocent ejaculators' into the mix and this number seems plausible.**

I want to surrender and so I'm going to make it happen. We try to force the issue—we try to impose our will on our body. This approach won't work—it's self-defeating. To become skilled at surrendering, we need to intend in a less yang way. We need to have faith in ourselves—and in the process, too. Our intending needs to be as soft and yin as the surrendering we're inviting our body to do. We have to surrender in both mind and body.

This is not to suggest there's no place for yang energy in the ejaculation process. As I've said, I've had many intensely yang ejaculations. When you give birth, you say yes to the process and then push out a baby. This is an intensely muscular activity. It's the same with squirting: You surrender and can then push out the fluid. You can be yang on top of yin.

Surrendering energetically is a very vulnerable experience. You need to feel safe to do it. Here are some of the chief obstacles that can make this difficult:

- You may have a history of sexual trauma, abuse or sexual shame.
- You may be with a partner who has a history of treating you inconsiderately or who isn't in tune with you emotionally. Or perhaps you're with a new partner you don't feel totally comfortable with yet. (This is why it can be easier to practice on your own.)
- You may be feeling inadequate because you 'should' be able to ejaculate like those women in porn.
- When the G-spot is being stimulated, emotions can arise that need to be processed or released. These embodied feelings can make it difficult to let go.

There are also more local and immediate concerns. Some women worry that their ejaculate may actually be urine and are horrified at the thought of peeing in the bed. Other women know their ejaculate isn't urine, but have compunctions about drenching the sheets and mattress anyway.

There are easy fixes for these logistical anxieties. First and foremost: Ladies, ejaculate isn't pee! Really and truly, it's not. As for the equally understandable fear of flooding, this is easily dealt with by purchasing waterproof pads. You can buy ones that are made for babies (little elephants, now that's sexy!). Put a bath towel on top of it and you're good to gush. You can also find special velvety machine-washable blankets that are specifically designed for female ejaculators. They're not cheap, but they do a great job of protecting the bed (or floor, or back of the Chevy).

Ejaculators-in-training, I can't stress enough the importance of creating an environment where you feel truly safe. This may include having a lover present and it may not. If you're at all concerned about mess, lay out a towel or waterproof blanket ahead of your session. When it comes to the learning process, don't 'should' on yourself. Take deep, slow breaths. Relax and then relax some more. Still your mind as best you can. Speak mantras of safety to yourself. Give yourself full permission to let go and fully experience what's there without a goal. The more you can stay connected to your body and all its sensations without getting lost in your head, the more you'll be able to let go and surrender. Eventually it will come.

And then there's the physical aspect of squirting. Spend lots of time with your G-spot. Since this is the part of the female erectile network that fills with ejaculate, when you stimulate your urethral sponge you're being hands-on in the most direct way possible.

Also pay lots of attention to the area immediately behind the sponge. See what happens when your or someone else's fingers are placed in that little declivity and do a 'come-hither' motion that brings the digits into contact with the back side of the sponge. This is the #1 pleasure spot for many women.

As I mentioned earlier, the G-spot is often a storehouse for emotions, including difficult ones. If you've been sexually abused or have experienced any kind of sexual trauma, a lot of your pain may be lodged there. I encourage you to spend a lot of quality time getting intimate with your G-spot. If painful emotions surface, let them happen. Remind yourself that you're releasing held energy and this means you're taking good care of yourself. Immense pleasure can await you on the other side of emotional pain.

Sometimes the G-spot has very little or no sensation when stimulated. If this is your situation, don't worry—the G-spot can increase in sensitivity as you give it more attention and stimulation. Don't give up because there weren't fireworks when you tried stimulating your G-spot the first time. It's amazing how sensitive the G-spot can become over time.

Toys can be a great aid if you're playing solo. Many women find it awkward or uncomfortable to spend extended amounts of time with their fingers inside themselves. G-spotter toys do a great job of hitting the spot (literally!), and they keep you comfortable while you're doing it.

Penises tend to be less effective than toys or fingers at directly stimulating the G-spot—they're a blunt instrument, relatively speaking, and most don't have the ideal 45° angle that a G-spotter toy or bent finger has. There are sexual positions that can maximize G-spot contact with a penis, though. Have fun finding them!

Next up on the anatomical hit parade is the clitoris. The G-spot and clit feed off each other and are entirely complementary. I think of the clitoris as the engine and the G-spot as the throttle. Clitoral stimulation combined with simultaneous G-spot stimulation is often a magical recipe for producing female ejaculation.

It's also possible to ejaculate from clitoral stimulation alone. Try playing with one, then the other, then put the two together and see how that feels.

The urethral opening (sometimes called the U-spot) is a sadly neglected piece of female genital anatomy. As we've seen, the urethral sponge is made up of erectile tissue, and it's also where ejaculate is produced. What many people tend to overlook is that the sponge can be accessed externally as well as internally. When the sponge is engorged, the lightest flick of a finger or tongue at the urethral opening is sometimes all it takes to get a body to gush.

I've spent a lot of time in these pages stressing the importance of surrendering. Now I'm going to discuss the other, yang side of the coin. For many women, the orgasmic experience is characterized by contraction. Things get tight; they pull in. When you're learning to ejaculate, you may want to practice getting comfortable with a different orgasmic experience. As you're coming, bear down and push out with your pelvic floor muscles. Doing this can encourage the release of fluid. Again, there's an analogy here to birthing. You're surrendering at one level and pushing down and out at another.

A key to ejaculating is surrendering to the process—letting it unfold.

Many women also find it helpful to remove anything that's inside the vagina as the moment of ejaculation approaches. You often see this in squirt porn. The penis or toy is pulled out and gushing follows immediately.

While I can testify to the effectiveness of this move, I'm less certain about why this is so. I do have a theory, though. When you have something inside you pressing up against the urethral sponge, it's being compressed—it's like a balloon full of air that's being squeezed. When you remove the pressure, there's suddenly room for expansion and the sponge fills with that much more ejaculate. This sudden shift takes you over the top—the liquid spills into the urethra and from there out into the world.

If there were a rote, paint-by-the-numbers way to get women to gush, that's what I'd be teaching. But there isn't. Women's sexuality is variable and so are their paths to ejaculating. The best I can offer is a suite of tools and suggestions. I encourage you to experiment and discover what works best for you. Between U-sponge play, clitoral stimulation, U-spot stimulation, bearing down and pushing out, and removing internal objects as ejaculation approaches, I'm confident you'll find the combination that transforms you into a gushing goddess.

And remember, always, the importance of safety and surrender.

Women's Two Biggest Challenges

Women face two main challenges when it comes to learning to ejaculate. The first is ignorance. They don't know ejaculation is possible, and if they do, they don't know how to make it happen.

Since you've gotten this far in this chapter, that's not you. The second challenge may apply to you, though. It's much easier to ejaculate if you're very deeply aroused. Improbable as it may seem, many women have never actually had this experience. In fact, because full female arousal is modeled virtually nowhere in our culture, they don't even know they're missing out! Few people know about the female erectile network (see Chapter One) or how to make it very happy.

Women, it's important to get your entire erectile network nice and juicy before putting anything inside you. Ideally, you'll stimulate all the network's components: the clitoral tip, shaft and legs, the vestibular bulbs, the perineal sponge and the G-spot. And remember: If you've got a penis, toy or fingers in your vagina and it doesn't feel great, remove said object(s) immediately. They shouldn't be there.

I encourage you to study up on full female arousal. Ejaculation and arousal go together like, well, a G-spotter toy in a well-primed, very juicy and engorged pussy.

Ejaculation as Affirmation

I don't need to say this but I will: Learning to squirt is entirely optional. You can have amazing sexual pleasure without being an ejaculator, and you can also be great in bed. A scarcity mindset should never be what drives you to become a gushing goddess. Let what you can be, not what you believe you lack, be your inspiration.

Also remember to have fun with it! Being light-hearted, experimental and open-minded throughout your journey will keep your juices flowing.

When I ejaculate, I don't just tap into the spirit of the divine feminine, I become the divine feminine. My mind lets go. My heart and spirit open. My body experiences amazing pleasure.

The experience is, among other things, a profound affirmation. When I'm in that wave of surrendering, I'm saying "Yes!" to an archetypal energy that's vastly more powerful than any single man or woman could possibly be. I'm riding a hot, ecstatic, perfect wave of what was, what is and what will be.

It's a heavenly experience. I recommend it heartily.

SEXY SUMMARY

JUST ABOUT EVERY WOMAN can learn to ejaculate.

FEMALE EJACULATE is produced inside the urethral sponge on the roof of the vagina. It's probably made up of blood plasma plus glandular material.

WOMEN'S SEXUALITY VARIES and their path to ejaculation varies, too. Simultaneous clitoris and sponge stimulation and playing with the urethral sponge internally and/or externally are two great options.

A KEY TO EJACULATING is learning to surrender.

IT'S ALSO IMPORTANT to have the erectile network fully aroused.

FEMALE EJACULATION can be a spiritually and emotionally transformative experience.

JAELEEN BENNIS *is the creator of Bondassage®, a program that licenses practitioners around the world in her uniquely sensual and provocative method of bodywork. She is a certified massage therapist (CMT) trained in shiatsu, deep tissue, Swedish and sports massage, and has studied cross-cultural healing modalities from Reiki to shamanic journeying. She is versed in Tantra and BDSM, and believes in sexual exploration as a path to self-discovery and healing.*

Bondassage

by Jaeleen Bennis & Carl Frankel

BONDASSAGE®, A CONCEPT I DEVELOPED IN 2008, COMES OUT OF my work as a massage therapist and professional dominant. While elements of domination are involved, as the name suggests it's really more about massage combined with bondage. It's a way to play with sensation—to enhance sensation, really, by adding the feelings of vulnerability and helplessness that come with a loss of control.

This loss of control comes from two things, bondage and sensory deprivation.

As a professional massage therapist, I adapted my massage table to accommodate the bondage part. I bought eye bolts and washers and drilled eight tie-down holes in the side of my table. This gives me many different positions for tying a person down. You don't need a customized massage table, or even an unmodified one, to do Bondassage, though. You can use a bed, the floor, or whatever works for you and your partner, so long as you're both comfortable. This is about pleasure, and although the focus is more on the receiver's pleasure than the giver's, it's important that neither of you be distracted by chafed wrists, hurting knees or whatever. This is why I use a massage table and it's also why I restrain *gently.* Bondassage involves creating a sense of powerlessness. While actual physical restraints help to drive the point home, the state of mind is ultimately more important than the reality. Use pretend cuffs if you want to.

When I'm doing a session, I like to have my receiver kneel and submit to being 'formally' cuffed and collared. This is entirely optional, though. You're trying to induce a mood of submission in your bottom. If a ritual helps, go for it.

And then there's sensory deprivation. As a species, we use our senses to spot dangers and opportunities. We rely heavily on our vision (that tiger in the tree!) and, to a lesser extent, our hearing (that rustling in the brush). If we can't use our senses, it makes us feel more vulnerable and exposed. There's nothing we can do about this—it's evolution's programming.

As a Bondassage practitioner, I tap into this ancient programming by temporarily relieving my receiver of the ability to see and hear what's occurring around them. I cover their eyes with a blindfold or scarf, and I pipe music into their ears through headphones. Some of my practitioners use a splitter so that their bottom hears the music through headphones but it's also being piped directly into the room. That way, the top also hears the music and can harmonize what they're doing with the receiver's listening experience.

Tied down (lightly), unable to see and unable to hear anything but trance-inducing music, the receiver is stripped of control, naked (both literally and figuratively) and, inevitably, acutely alert. All sensations are magnified because the receiver can't predict, much less control, what's coming next.

I'm transporting my bottom into a trance state. I'm taking them on a trip, and I'm steering with sensation.

Before the Fun Begins

Before any of that, though, like every good Boy Scout, you'll want to be prepared. This means talking to your partner about their likes, dislikes and limits. If you're going to be doing food play, ask about allergies! Anaphylactic shock isn't fun or sexy.

Many people have very strong reactions to smells. Before you collar them, check in about what smells and tastes they love and which they can't tolerate.

The 'check-in' principle also applies to other kinds of sensation. If someone gets squicked out by a Wartenberg wheel—a toy like a miniature pizza wheel that's used in kinky play—you don't want to be surprising them with it when they're blindfolded and helpless on the table.

You can get all this information without sacrificing the important element of surprise. Your check-in will give you a general sense of what will enhance and detract from your bottom's experience. You'll still have a lot of room for improvisation within those boundaries.

I'm not a big fan of setting time limits. If you agree to do a session for, say, one hour, that puts pressure on the top to come up with ways to fill the time. It gives the bottom a greater sense of control because they know when the session will end. In addition, hard time limits can keep the top from getting into creative flow. Maybe you'll get into exploring all the things you can do with a feather duster and when you look up, an hour and a half has gone by. You don't want your trance cut short by an arbitrary time limit.

That said, people do have real-world obligations. If your partner has to pick up the kids at four o'clock, you'll probably want to establish in advance that you need to wrap up the session by 3:30.

If you wish, you can outfit your space with sex furniture that will enhance the Bondassage experience. One company sells ramps and wedges that make it easy to put your receiver into a comfortable and erotically convenient and arousing position. Their products include wedges and ramps with straps attached for wrist and ankle cuffs. (Details are in the Resources section.)

There's no need to go out and buy special furniture, though. A standard bed or massage table works on its own just fine, and if you're inclined to try something else, conventional furniture will often do the trick. I use an inexpensive rocking chair for bondage.

For massage, though, you'll want to have a stable, comfortable, padded surface.

Gather your props in advance—while pauses can be sexy, the extended delay that occurs while you go downstairs for that rubber spatula you forgot is just boring and annoying. Organize your goodies so you can easily lay your hands on what you're looking for. You're the top and not only do you want to project a sense of authority, you also want to feel that way internally. A surgeon knows where their tools are. So does a skilled Bondassage practitioner.

I go into each session with a beginner's mind. I know how I'm going to begin and I make a point of having my tools and toys available, but after that I just try to stay present and be guided by the cues my receiver gives me.

Making Sensation Sensational

Once my bottom has, so to speak, assumed the position, I start with a massage. Three distinct types of touch are usually involved—therapeutic, which has healing as its purpose; sensual, which is intended to be pleasing; and erotic, which is sexually arousing. For me, erotic touch includes genital, anal and internal touch along with breast and nipple massage, but it does not include oral play or intercourse. I'm not saying you can't do the latter during Bondassage, just that for me they're not 'massage.'

The categories can overlap. You can do therapeutic massage in a sensual manner by slowing down or by intending to touch sensually. You can sprinkle erotic touch into sensual.

In your session, you can try alternating these modalities or, if you prefer, follow a progression from therapeutic through sensual to erotic. There are no rules here: Bondassage is an improvisation. Do what feels right based on intuition and, more importantly, the signals you get from your receiver.

You can use different parts of your body to give a massage. Fingers, the center of the palm (which I call the 'heart') and the heel of the hand are obvious candidates. Elbows and knuckles are great for going deep. Hair can be fun and breasts can be a big winner no matter what size they are. If you're a penis owner, you can use your equipment to do sensual or erotic touch, although bear in mind that your goal is to take the receiver on a journey into ecstasy, not to go there yourself. You're the guide here, not the traveler.

I usually include some percussion in my sensation play—spanking, slapping and such. I keep it all very light, though. As a professional dominatrix, if someone wants pain, I know how to give it. That's not where I go with Bondassage, though, and I don't recommend it. Bondassage is about sensation, not pain. Floggers and canes can stimulate and arouse without hurting.

This is a crucially important point. *Bondassage is not about pain.* This isn't to say that the sensations can't be very intense, or that it can't involve experiences that would be painful if the receiver weren't aroused. A nipple tweak, for instance, can hurt if you're not turned on yet be delicious if you are. As a rule, though, you don't want to be adding pain to the sensation potpourri unless your receiver specifically requests it.

During a given Bondassage session, I might use two or three different percussion instruments, maybe a flogger and some canes, which as I said I use really lightly. I like Wartenberg wheels and like to experiment with objects that can be found around the house. I'm especially fond of vibrating electric toothbrushes, which I use as a brush without power or fire up and use the bristles or back as a vibrator.

I call toys like these "pervertibles." Which makes Costco, Home Depot and Bed, Bath and Beyond some of the best sex stores in the world! The kitchen aisles are especially full of opportunities.

There's a lesson here beyond the entertainment value. Be creative!

Less is more in Bondassage. I encourage practitioners to choose a couple of toys and dive deeply into them rather than have fifty things on their table. Too much variety can come across as random and chaotic. Also, you don't want to be thinking about the five things you'll be doing next—you want to be present to what you're doing now. Beginners make this mistake a lot. They go out and cobble together the 750 things they want to play with, then it's two seconds of this and three seconds of that and it all comes across as disjointed.

Bondassage is not about pain.

You can do a lot with very little. I once did an entire session using only a wooden hairbrush. I dragged the bristles along the body and used them for percussion. I used the smooth sides and back for stroking. I put a condom on the handle and used it internally. It was fun for me and my receiver loved every minute of it.

A Sampling of Pervertibles

Hot

Wax
Hot water (use eye dropper)
Cayenne pepper
Ginger
Hot breath
Tiger Balm
Warm washcloth
Hand warmers for skiing

Cold

Ice
Chain
Pearls
Ice cups
Ice cubes
Polar Lotion/Icy Hot
Canned air spray

Soft

Rabbit fur
Feathers
Satin
Silk scarf
Paint brush
Makeup brush
Silicone basting brushes

Pinchy

Clothespins
Clips
Clamps
Plastic vise grips
Alligator clips

Scratchy

Forks
Bottle caps
Metal hair brushes
Whisks
Toothpicks
Combs
Fingernails
Brush
Pipecleaners
Loofah

Suction

Snakebite kit
Cupping sets

Vibration

Disposable electric toothbrushes
TENS unit
Vibrator

Smell

Essential oils
Flowers
Pine branches
Citrus
Vanilla
Cinnamon

Taste (and Smell)

Popsicles
Chocolate
Honey
Jam
Whipped cream
Breath mints
Flavored lip gloss

I encourage you not to follow a script. It takes the fun and spontaneity out to 'top by numbers.' You want to be present and go with the flow of what's happening, and this is likeliest to happen if you come into the session with a few props and a lot of creativity.

Taste and smell experiences are great additional ways to play. What you're doing with Bondassage is exploring the range of physical sensations, so why not add taste and scent to the menu? Once a person is in a highly aroused state—and this may or may not mean sexually aroused—being given something delicious to taste can tip them into ecstasy. I've seen people have energy orgasms from having their lips rubbed with chocolate.

Do think things through first, though. If you're working with taste, you might want to pre-plan a sequence, almost as if you were designing a meal at a fine restaurant. Peanut butter is probably not a great way to start because the taste and texture will linger. Moving among the main flavor groups of sweet, savory, salty and spicy can be a fun way to proceed. You can organize this by taking an empty ice tray and putting different taste samples in each cube container.

You can also experiment with essential oil diffusers, switching out scents in the course of a session.

One practitioner friend of mine likes to crush or rub oregano under her receiver's nose when they're at the point of orgasm. She does this because, in her words, "Now when they're in pizza parlors, they'll think of me." While this pervy little pleasure won't be for everyone, it's worth noting for two reasons. First, it reminds us how individual and personalized you can make the experience. Second, it encourages practitioners to be ambitious—why not strive to create a truly memorable experience?

I encourage you, like my oregano-wielding friend, to develop your own signature. Chocolate truffles are mine. At the end of a session, my receiver is usually pretty tranced out. When they start to emerge, I ask them if they can eat chocolate and, if the answer is yes, if they prefer light or dark. Then I pop a truffle in their mouth. It's a lovely way to welcome them back to mundane reality.

Bondassage sessions can be followed by sex . . . or not. They can include sexual touching . . . or not. They can include an orgasm . . . or not. There are no rules here other than what the participants agree to. When we train people to do Bondassage, we teach four endings—the giver helps the receiver have an orgasm, the receiver self-pleasures to orgasm, the receiver is denied an orgasm, and the receiver is taken through what Taoists call the 'big draw.' As I learned this practice, you do thirty fast inhales and exhales through your mouth. This is followed by three long, deep breaths—in and hold, then exhale, another deep breath in followed by a hold and exhale, then a third time. On the third inhalation, you clench all your muscles as tightly as you can—toes, anus, hands, mouth and everything in between. You do this for as long as you can and then you let go. The body lifts off into a blissful state that feels orgasmic but isn't ejaculatory.

Please Don't Just Lie There

As a top, it can be unsettling to be doing all kinds of wonderful things to your bottom and have them lie there without reacting. All kinds of doubts of the "I must be doing something wrong" variety can rush into that silence. While it's natural to want to get something back from your bottom, it's important to remember that silence doesn't necessarily signify unhappiness. I learned this from a client who was initially mute and unexpressive and then, during the post-session aftercare, told me, "I was screaming inside my head."

I encourage tops to ask their bottoms to communicate what's going on for them—not necessarily in words, which can undermine the trance state, but with sound and body movement. You do want the bottom to relax and let go—you don't want them feeling like they need to perform for you—but it's also okay to request (or even require) certain behaviors from them. If you tell them that giving feedback will help you pleasure them better, that makes for a pretty compelling argument.

The reality is that some people get self-conscious and have trouble making sound. Headphones and a blindfold can help here. They shift the context for the bottom—it's as if their sound is being projected somewhere that has nothing to do with them. This makes vocalizing easier.

Of course, it can be easy to tell if men are enjoying the experience. Erections are a great barometer. Even then, though, it can enhance the top's experience for the bottom to give voice to their pleasure. An erection signifies general, non-specific approval. Moans and sighs—and their absence—tell the top that this move is working really well, that move not so much.

Keys to Doing Bondassage Well

Ultimately, Bondassage is about trust. The receiver can't totally surrender to sensation and pleasure if they're not totally confident that their top is going to take good care of them. It's important to establish this relationship at the start and not betray it. This is done in numerous ways. There's the pre-session conversation about boundaries, likes, dislikes and allergies. There's the initial submission ritual, where the bottom, in kneeling and accepting the collar, says symbolically, "I trust you enough to hand my power over to you." There's the session itself, when the giver starts off slow and light and pays exquisite attention to the receiver and their responses. And, finally, there's aftercar wind-down, when the receiver gets loving attention from their dominant. I mean, really—does anything say it like chocolate?

I'll add what may already be obvious to you. The submissive isn't really handing their power over to their dominant. This is play, a game that can be called off at any time by the bottom or the top. It's a relationship between equals where one person agrees to be the giver and the other agrees to be the receiver. Ultimately it's the bottom who's in control because they're the one who establishes the boundaries and can call an end to the game at will.

Your Prime Directives here are comfort and pleasure, mostly for the bottom but for the top as well. As I've mentioned, I'm a big fan of headphones for the auditory experience. They pump up the quality of the bottom's experience by orders of magnitude. I use wireless headphones that cost about $100 online. They're cushy and comfortable and provide an adequate audio experience.

Some of my practitioners have splurged on high-end wired headphones, and while that creates great sound, the wires can get in the way.

Over the years, I've experimented with different headphone brands. I once used a model with an AM/FM receiver that suddenly switched over to a baseball game in the middle of a session. This did not enhance the experience although my team was winning.

I use music with a slow groove that is either entirely instrumental or in a language my bottom can't understand. Comprehensible words keep people in their head and I want my receivers to get out of their heads and into body awareness.

Once you're set up, start slowly. And softly. Your bottom's experience of sensation is intensified and you don't want to shock or overstimulate them by doing too much too soon. Don't worry about not providing a compelling experience—slow and soft can feel wonderful at any time, and at the beginning of a session they'll be more pleasing than fast and hard. Consider using something like a satin pillow case, fleece or piece of fur to rub all over your receiver's body.

If I could give practitioners only one piece of advice, it would be this: Slow down—and then slow down some more. It will intensify your bottom's experience, and it will also help you tune in better make fewer mistakes. Go slowly and pay close attention to how your receiver is responding. Gradually build the intensity.

It's also important to touch skilfully. While the quality of touch always matters in a massage session, it's especially true with Bondassage because the receiver is in such a highly sensitized state. When doing therapeutic touch, I tend to use a firm surface like my elbows, a stiff palm or my fingers, and I apply firm pressure.

While sensual and erotic touch differ in important ways, I do both using the heart of my palm as my touch 'center.' Depending on my purpose, I visualize sending heart or erotic energy into my receiver through my palm—it becomes a conduit, essentially. Same palm, different intentions. That's not all I touch with, of course—I also use my fingertips, the back of my hands, my fingernails and my whole hand for sensual and erotic massage, and other body parts like my breasts for erotic massage—but in terms of energy and focus, the heart of my palm is my baseline. It's my starting point—it's where I center, where I put my energy—and then I let my hand and fingers relax and get soft around it. For instance, if I'm doing clitoral massage, I might press the center of my palm on my receiver's pubic bone and drape my fingers over her vulva. That way, I'm feeling the connection through the center of my palm and then letting that awareness radiate out through my fingers.

Kinesthetic intelligence—the ability to be present through touch—varies from person to person. It's like IQ in the sense that some people have more and some have less. But unlike IQ, touch is something you can learn. With practice, anyone can learn to touch skilfully, including those who come to the (massage) table without special gifts in that area. There is a technical aspect to skillful touch, but it's secondary. First, you need to be able to get out of your head and into your fingers—you need to be present in a way that's very different from what our usual busy-brain duties require. Once you move your consciousness into your fingers, you'll often find that your kinesthetic intelligence awakens and you're more much intuitively attuned than you believed you could be.

Slow down. And then slow down some more.

Touch is an ability that can be cultivated. And Bondassage is a great way to do it.

Why Do Bondassage?

Bondassage is catching on fast. Why? Timing has a lot to do with it—kink is going mainstream and Bondassage is 'kink-esque.' It's also sexy and fun, and a great way for people who are new to kink to play with dominance and submission and learn more about impact play.

Power play is frequently misunderstood and misapplied by beginners. Newbies often associate being dominant with being harsh or unkind. This is fine if it turns the bottom on, but it's not required. BDSM is also often associated with pain, and that needn't be the case either. Because Bondassage doesn't have these associations, it doesn't encourage these mistakes. It's 'domination light,' and for this reason a great framework for people who are just getting started with kink.

Bondassage can be a great confidence-builder for the top because when your receiver is strapped down and can neither see nor hear you, they're not going to see you fumbling around with the ropes or turning stuff upside-down looking for the next toy on your playlist. In fact, sensory deprivation doesn't only keep them from judging your performance, it also heightens their anticipation and turn-on. It's a win-win for you both.

And, remember, stillness and silence can be 'moves' in their own right.

More broadly, Bondassage offers participants a way to become more skilled erotically. It helps both givers and receivers learn to be more present, which is probably the first key to being a great lover. As the top, you need to pay exquisitely close attention to your bottom. You notice their breath, their sound and the motions their bodies make. You notice how aroused they are and whether they want more of the same or less. Are they arching their buttocks up to request more spanking? Are they clenching their cheeks and trying to get away from you? You also need to pay attention to how you touch, whether it's with your own body parts or with tools and toys.

As the bottom, Bondassage teaches you to let go and surrender to sensation. The deeper you can go into an altered state, the more sublime your experience will be. Getting out of your head isn't only a way to have more fun, it's also an erotic skill. The more you can learn to go deeply into your trance, the better you'll be at both receiving and giving pleasure.

Bondassage is a fun, fascinating way to connect sensually and erotically. It makes wonderful foreplay and is a great canvas for improvisation.

It's a fine framework for developing your overall erotic skills and refining your skills as a top or bottom.

It's a way to take a grand mind-bending trip without ever leaving home. Or taking drugs.

Now get out there and gather those pervertibles!

SEXY SUMMARY

Bondassage is a type of sensation play that works with a perceived loss of control in the receiver. This loss of control comes from two things, bondage and sensory deprivation.

Trust is critically important and needs to be established at every stage of the session.

Pain is optional and at the sole discretion of the receiver.

While you'll want to bring structure into your session, make sure you also leave room for creativity and improvisation.

Receivers, you'll probably have a better experience if you communicate actively with your giver.

Bondassage is a great way to learn touch skills and to play with 'kink light.'

CHARLES MUIR *is considered the originator and pioneer of the modern Tantra movement in the United States. In 1980, he originated the Tantra: The Art of Conscious Loving® format, Sacred Spot Massage, and many other inventive experiential exercises that have become cornerstones in the curriculum of many Tantra educators. He is the founder of the Source School of Tantra Yoga.*

In addition to Red Tantra practices, Charles teaches a powerful method of White Tantra, or Laya Yoga, which is the grandfather of Hatha Yoga, with extended holds, meditation, and chakra focus. Its gentle-on-the-body approach is relaxing and revitalizing, and awakens consciousness quickly.

Charles has authored two Tantra books, two Tantra Training DVDs, three White Tantra CDs, and five Red Tantra CDs. His work has been featured in over fifty media articles, numerous radio and television appearances (most recently on Oprah*), and two Hollywood feature movies,* Bliss *and* The Best Ever. *He is currently working on several new books in his Tantra: The Art of Conscious Loving series—the newest is* Sacred Sexual Awakenings, *which is a comprehensive compilation of over five hundred testimonials and case histories of lives transformed through attending his seminars.*

Charles has been quoted in over 130 books on Tantra, relationship and yoga. He has trained over 200 teachers worldwide in his unique Tantra Sexuality format.

Source Tantra's website is SourceTantra.com, where you will find over 60 free instructional videos and 40 media articles. His e-mail address is charles@sourcetantra.com.

CHAPTER SIXTEEN

Tantra

by Charles Muir & Carl Frankel

FOUR DECADES AGO, HARDLY ANYONE IN THE WEST HAD HEARD OF Tantra, a set of esoteric sexual practices developed in India several millennia ago. Things are different now, thanks in large part to Sting. And the Internet. In the early 1990s, word got out that he often made love to his wife for five hours and more in a single session using Tantric techniques. It's an urban legend—Sting was making a joking response in an interview to a throwaway line by fellow musician Bob Geldof about his being a three-minute man—but no matter: Sting will be known forever as a super-lover whose magical abilities owe everything to Tantra.

Forget 'be like Mike.' Can we agree that what men really want is to be like Sting?

As Tantra has made its way into the public domain, its meaning has sometimes been distorted. Thousands of years ago, sacred prostitutes offered themselves sexually in the context of religious worship. In one recent instance, an enterprising entrepreneur opened an enterprise that promoted itself as offering sacred massage using what were labeled 'Tantra techniques.' She wasn't running a bordello, it was a 'temple.' Customers didn't pay for services, they offered a donation, the same way you would when the donation box comes around at church on Sunday morning.

This wasn't Tantra. It was a rub-and-tug with some breathing techniques thrown in.

Here's another way Tantra is sometimes misrepresented. Individual facets are taught without reference to the whole. I know people who teach sacred-spot massage, which is a single Tantra technique, and call it Tantra. It's not—it's like a single toe on a vast body of learning. Tantra is a complex, sophisticated body of knowledge and practice, not a grab-bag of sex tricks.

Having spent the last forty years of my life learning and teaching Tantra, I'm delighted that it's going mainstream. I'm less thrilled at the extent to which the concept is cheapened by its associations with fame and ego ("Screw like Sting!") and pseudo-spirituality ("Our happy endings bring you close to God"). Tantra is a powerful, serious (and seriously fun!) series of techniques that require study and mastery. While Tantra does involve sexual activity, the ultimate goal isn't to become great in bed or even to dissolve the boundaries between you and your partner. It's to experience union with the Beloved within.

And it just so happens that along the way, you encounter your partner's divinity, you become really skilled in bed, and you experience levels of ecstasy that far exceed what you can get with your usual sex, delightful though that is.

The purpose of Tantra is to achieve union with the Beloved within.

Many people I know have taken up meditation as a spiritual practice. They had great intentions but could never quite find the time to sit in stillness. Then they switched to Tantra and found themselves practicing nightly for hours. Fun, delight and ecstasy are great motivators. When a person discovers how amazing sex can be, it's as if they've eaten fast food all their life and are dining in a gourmet French restaurant for the first time. Once you discover how great food nourishes you energetically, spiritually, physically and psychologically, take-out burgers won't hold much luster any more.*

You know how there are 'friends with benefits?' Well, Tantra is a spiritual practice with benefits.

Tantra Defined

As we've seen, Tantra isn't just a way to have sex. It's a type of yoga. In fact, the full name for Tantra is Tantra yoga. 'Tantra' is an abbreviation—it's sort of like calling Joseph 'Joe.'

In the west, yoga is usually associated with stretching exercises and Tantra with sex. While somewhat accurate, these associations are also a bit misleading because they disregard all the other components of the practice as well as the ultimate goal of these activities—they confuse the means with the end. Yoga's purpose isn't to help people become limber and Tantra's isn't to help them have great sex. It's to unify the partners' energies so that the sum of

---

*** I'm not knocking the sort of sex most people have. It's a way for people to connect and be loving, it's fun, it's a great way to make babies if that's what you want to do, and it can also feel really good. It also gets some people launched on a path toward more ecstatic loving.**

their energy is greater than its parts, a sort of energetic big bang results, and it takes them to a place of transcendent, ecstatic bliss.

Some etymology may be useful here. When outsiders think of yoga, they usually have hatha yoga in mind. Hatha's two syllables mean sun and moon, respectively. Yoga means 'yoking' or 'union.' Thus hatha yoga involves the union of the sun and the moon, or of the masculine and feminine energies. As for Tantra, 'tan' means expanding, in the sense that the universe is expanding. 'Tra' means weaving, like you do with a textile. Thus when we practice Tantra yoga, we weave together ('tra') energy in a way that brings us to a state of expanded consciousness ('tan') and enables us to achieve union with the Beloved within ('yoga').

It's also important to differentiate between White and Red Tantra yoga. White Tantra (or Laya yoga), which is the grandfather of Hatha yoga, is a solo practice. You get into a position that typically involves some sort of stretch and is based on sacred geometry, you regulate your breathing and focus your mind using meditation, and you learn how to stimulate the chakras while in these positions. (I'll say more about the chakras below.) When you do White Tantra, you're working with the masculine and feminine energies inside you. You're bringing them into a state of balance and unity by releasing blocked energy and consciousness.*

With Red Tantra, which is what people typically associate with Tantra, you're integrating outer male and female energies, which affect your inner masculine and feminine. You're practicing with a partner and it involves sex and other practices.

As I've said, Tantra is thousands of years old. As with anything that old and revered, there are lineages, which means that there are strict rules from one master or another about how to do Tantra, and these rules are passed down from generation to generation via anointed successors.

The Tantra I teach wasn't passed on to me by a single teacher. Over the years, I've learned from many people. Trial-and-error has been my path. I practiced the techniques and observed the results. If something didn't work particularly well for me, I tried something different. I recommend the same approach to my students. Personal experience is our best teacher.

My method has evolved into a lineage called Source Tantra. Over the years, I've initiated over 40,000 people into the mysteries of Tantra. I also have a certification program for people who want to teach Source Tantra.

*** 'Masculine and feminine energy' is not the same as male and female body parts. We all have masculine and feminine within us. This is true regardless of our sexual preference or plumbing. Thus Tantra is for gay people as well as for heterosexuals.**

Tantra Techniques

In a chapter of this length, I can't possibly teach you Tantra. The best I can do is provide a taste of what you'll learn if you decide to study Tantra.

LOCATING AND MOVING ENERGY. One essential skill you'll develop is the ability to locate and move energy. When sexual energy is shut down, it affects us at every level of our psyche. Tantra students learn to identify where their partner's sexual energy is blocked or sluggish—it usually shows up as an area of physical tenderness. Let's say you're with a woman who's been out of her marriage for a year and is just starting to date. You sense that her heart is shut down. You want to awaken this energy—you want to bring her heart, her capacity to feel love, alive again. If this were your goal, you'd touch her heart and breasts very differently than if you were seeking to arouse her (and yourself) sexually.

ACTIVATING THE CHAKRAS. The word 'chakra' means 'wheel' in Sanskrit and refers to energy centers in the body, as identified by the Hindu and other spiritual traditions. While different systems name and locate them differently, the most widely accepted version has seven different energy centers, or chakras. In most people, some of these chakras are blocked and others aren't. The throat chakra, or voice, may be blocked. The second chakra, or sex center, may be shut down. Or maybe it's the heart that's not open. In my experience, many people who've done a lot of meditation have their higher chakras (from the heart and above) open, but their lower chakras, which involve the gritty 'non-spiritual' topics of survival, sex and power, are blocked.

One of the central goals of Tantra is to activate and align all seven chakras so they're flowing freely, powerfully and harmoniously. Aligning the upper and lower chakras is what brings us into a state of dynamic wholeness and spiritual awakening. It's what enables us to experience abundance. We support this process by teaching people how to tune into chakra energy and work with it.

In my earlier example, the woman's heart chakra has been shut down by the collapse of her marriage. The energy that comes out of your hands is an extension of your own heart chakra. Once you've identified her emotional and energetic blockage, you can imprint your own energy with loving feelings along with the intention to help her heart chakra open. One option would be to cup her breasts and nipples with the palms of your hands and use your fingers to touch the center line of her body between her breasts, which is the heart chakra line. Doing this often brings the psychic pain to the surface and results in emotional release. Tantra students learn to go to their partner's stuck energy places and move their blocked energy.

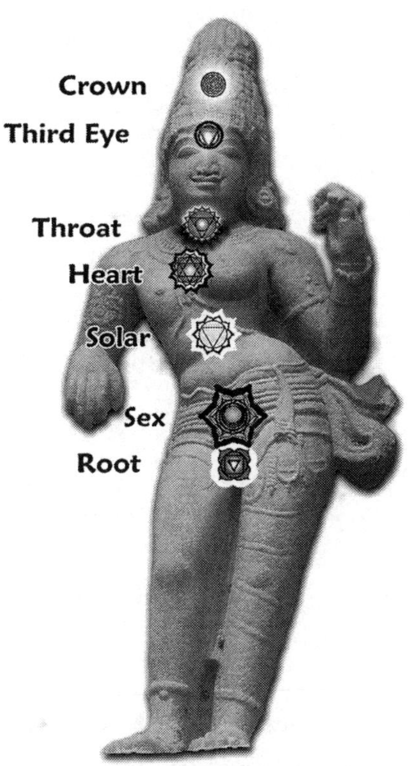

The Chakras
(art by Sheri Winston)

While your touch in this example is therapeutic, it's also foreplay. It's just not erotic foreplay—if you wanted to arouse her sexually, you'd caress her breasts more actively. By helping her release blocked energy, you're making it possible to connect more powerfully on an energetic level. This makes your erotic connection that much more explosive when the time comes to be directly sexual.

New Erogenous Zones. Another specialized Tantra skill involves the ability to identify erogenous zones. Knowing about the genitals, the neck and ear lobes, and the breasts in women is Foreplay 101. But the Tantra approach goes beyond this. For us, the chakra centers front and back are erogenous zones, and so we direct our attention—and energy— there. And because the flexible joints conduct lots of energy, they, too, are erogenous zones. We also put special attention there.

Quieting the Mind. Yet another Tantra skill is the ability to quiet the logical left hemisphere of the brain while activating the feeling, intuitive right hemisphere, which is where all mystical experience happens. What we're really doing here is activating our capacity to love because love is a mystical experience. We do this by altering our breathing. In beginner's seminars, we teach four types of breathing that affect relaxation levels, the ability to transmit and receive energy, and the duration of the orgasm.

Expanded Orgasm. The average orgasm for men lasts plus or minus ten seconds. Using specialized Tantra techniques, you can have orgasms that last five to ten breaths instead of seconds, with each breath lasting twenty seconds or longer. That's right: You can have orgasms lasting well beyond a minute. The key is to breathe in deeply as the orgasm begins, pulling the feeling of orgasmic energy upwards to the brain. Then you make sound on the exhalation. Sound opens the throat chakra, and opening the throat chakra on your exhale creates the downward flow of energy, or apana, that makes extended orgasm possible.

This technique enables both men and women to expand their orgasmic baseline, whatever that might be.

When people expand their orgasm using Tantra techniques, they're retraining their brain. We come into Tantra with certain assumptions about the orgasmic experience, such as the fact that if you're a guy, it ends pretty quickly. Tantra rewrites that story. An orgasm comes (so to speak) to mean something else.

Tantra is thus mind-expanding as well as orgasm-expanding. It opens us to a vastly more generous understanding of our capacity to experience ecstasy, and it also trains our brain to make traveling down the expanded-ecstasy highway our new normal. Tantra is thus profoundly transformational.

Sacred-Spot Massage. Another Tantra technique we teach is sacred-spot massage, which I mentioned earlier. There's a point inside both men and women's bodies called *yoni nadi* that can produce a super-intense sexual response—but it's not only sexual. It can also trigger emotional release accompanied by sexual healing.

The sacred spot is where people's psycho-sexual energy is stored. If that energy is blocked, it's where their blocked energy is held. These blocks may be due to conditioning, unresolved mother or father issues, or maybe the person was molested. There are many possible reasons. Because we all have 'stuff,' everyone can benefit from sacred-spot massage.

In women, the sacred spot is in the general area where the G-spot is located, though they're not identical. In men it can be activated through the perineum (the space between the testicles and the buttocks) or via the anus. Because it's associated with an energy center, not a single physical location, the sacred spot can actually move. It's here one moment, there the next. Tantra practitioners learn to find the sacred spot no matter where it's moved to.

When the sacred spot is massaged, it often results in a tremendous release of energy. It may be sexual, it may be emotional, and it's often spiritual.

The receiver may also feel numbness or even pain, depending on how their psycho-sexual energy is being held.

As with much of Tantra, the goal of sacred-spot massage isn't to produce orgasms, although that often happens. It's to help the receiver get in touch with themselves at a level where their awareness is usually repressed. This is done through a combination of technique and attitude. We teach nine sacred spot massage strokes. Some clear out blocks, others amp up sexual energy, and still others invite the receiver to go deep into their psyche.

It's important for both genders, and especially for men, to approach giving sacred-spot massage as nurturers. To surrender fully to the experience, women in particular need to be deeply trusting of their partner. This is likelier to happen if the giver holds space for her instead of just 'doing' her.

We encourage sacred-spot massage partners to approach the activity as a form of play. They'll do better as kids playing doctor than they will as doctors playing doctor. It's an exploration. An adventure.

STILLNESS. Another important Tantra technique is stillness. It's the exact opposite of what people usually want to do when things are going hot and heavy—the friction is the action, right? But there's enormous power in slowing down and, beyond that, in pausing. When you get still, you're replacing motion with attention—you're noticing what you're experiencing and opening new doorways to intimacy. This awareness alone can produce dramatic effects as you become more attuned to the energetics of what's occurring. Plus, things unfold in stillness that wouldn't happen if you were still grinding away. Things like waves of orgasmic pleasure. These aren't the sort of energy releases that will end the session if you're a man—they're a chapter in your ecstatic journey. You can go back to active lovemaking when the two of you are ready.

Tantra isn't just about creating pleasure. It's about creating love.

Underlying this advocacy of stillness is Tantra's commitment to balancing masculine and feminine energy. Ours is a culture of doing—it has a masculine bias in the sense that masculine 'yang' energy is associated with actively making things happen. While there's a place for this, there's also a place for stepping aside and letting things happen. When you get still, you're honoring feminine energy—you're being 'yin.' You're surrendering to the moment rather than trying to control it. The erotic payoff can be huge. When the energy 'does' you, it's an amazing experience.

Kissing. Yet another Tantra skill involves specific erotic techniques around kissing. There are energy meridians that run into the upper and lower lip. Tantra students learn how to tap these meridians because they send energy directly into the tip of the penis in men and the clitoris in women.

Sexual Positions. There are also recommendations around sexual positions. Each position creates a new energetic mandala, affecting the chakras in different ways.* We favor having the woman be on top more. It puts her more in control of her pleasure.

Penis Practices. Tantra also has specific recommendations for men regarding how to move their penis when they're inside their partner. Many men hump and pump just like they did as a teenager. Your penis doesn't need to be a blunt instrument. There are many different speeds and depths at which to move, and many different angles. Timing matters a lot here—there is a time for fast and hard and a time for slow and sensitive. There's also, as we've seen, the power of total stillness.

The reality is that you won't become a skilled ecstatic lover by relying on 'what comes naturally' or by watching porn. It takes study—and it also requires a new intention. Tantra isn't just about creating pleasure. It's about creating love.

More specifically, it's about working with energy to generate love. And it just so happens that sex is the vehicle for this.

Why and How to Learn Tantra

Anyone can learn Tantra so long as the commitment is there. My students come from all over the world and from every age group. At a recent seminar, three generations of the same family attended. The son bought his parents and his children and they all loved it. Many of the younger students are attracted by the hipper aspects of Tantra. They're drawn in by the Sting story and learn some of the techniques but focus less on the yoga. Others are touched by the quality and depth of the love that they see being generated. Or they note that Mom and Dad have become happier and more fulfilled since they started doing Tantra and decide they want to learn it, too.

You don't need to belong to an energy elite to learn Tantra. It's not for the specially gifted. We all have bodies; we all have energy centers; we all breathe. With practice, we can all learn how to do Tantra. I've had people

---

* *A mandala is a geometric symbol that awakens consciousness.*

A Sampling of Tantra Tools

Tune in with Spoons. "You don't have to wait for that magical moment when you're both in the mood," says Charles. Create the mood by getting in the spoon position, lying down, one holding the other from behind. Be still and synchronize your breathing. This puts you in tune with your partner.

Take Time Out. Here's a pause that expresses: When you're making love, stop moving for two minutes. Synchronize your breathing. Then hold your partner and look intently at each other. Imagine you are sending your energy back and forth as you synchronize your breathing. This exercise creates an even greater energy level and allows your lovemaking to be more emotional and less goal-oriented.

Keeping Abreast. "The breasts need to be touched, without being just a prelude to sex," says Caroline (my ex-wife). Heat up some scented lotion in the microwave or in your hands. Make gentle circles in the center of his chest. Ask your partner to touch his own breasts. Put your hands over his and learn how he wants to be touched. Have him do the same for you. Show him exactly how you love to be touched.

Touch Up Your Touch. Take five minutes each day to consciously touch your partner. Try to include these types of touch, varying the speed and intensity: Non-moving, caressing, circling, kneading, and gentle pinching, scratching and tapping. Bring love, nurturing and compassion into your touch.

From Tantra: The Art of Conscious Loving, by Charles and Caroline Muir *(Mercury House)*

---

with Asperger's Syndrome take my classes and despite their challenges with communication and empathy, they successfully learned it. They actually had cognitive breakthroughs, gaining better access to their feelings and becoming more skilled at communicating.

I noted earlier that Tantra carves out new neural pathways—it enables us to break away from old, routine and relatively narrow response patterns and to experience ourselves, our partners and the world as fundamentally more ecstatic. Some people let go of held emotional pain and are better able to experience life's positive aspects. A woman who couldn't have orgasms may become orgasmic. A woman who could only have clitoral orgasms may start having whole-body orgasms.

Every time you practice Tantra, you're refreshing yourself spiritually, emotionally, neurologically and biochemically. It's like taking a stagnant pool of water and running a fresh, crystal-clear stream through it. Because of this, some people speculate that Tantra and its cousin Taoism may ward off the cognitive decline that comes with aging. This is the view of the Taoist master Mantak Chia, who in a recent seminar commented that "science has proven" that ecstatic sex helps prevent Alzheimer's. I don't know what study he was referring to, but the proposition makes sense logically. If you're constantly moving energy up through your skull and carving out new ecstatic pathways, it stands to reason that your brain will stay fresh and won't rust, so to speak.

If you're feeling the urge to learn Tantra, what are your next steps? You can read about Tantra (see the Resources section). At the end of the day, though, you can only learn Tantra by doing. You've got to get out of your head and into your body, and practice the techniques. This is best done with the help of a skilled teacher.

You'll need to do some homework to find a good mentor. If you live in Boston, google 'Tantra teacher Boston' and see who comes up. But be cautious: This is unregulated territory. Anyone can put up a shingle and claim to be a Tantra teacher—the law won't come down on them. Do your due diligence. Have they written on the subject? Do they have YouTube videos and are they compelling? Do they have their own website? How long have they been teaching? What do other students say about them? Do they have some sort of credible certification? If they've been certified by me as a Certified Tantra Educator (CTE), that's a pretty good indication that they know what they're doing, though bear in mind that I have multiple levels of certification, so some of my certified teachers will be more skilled and knowledgeable than others.

I also recommend joining a Tantra community. This doesn't require you to have sex with lots of people, although some Tantra practitioners do—many Tantra practitioners have a very generous notion of what it means to "share the love." Whether you practice with only your partner or with others too, being part of a group deepens and accelerates the learning experience.

* * *

I love Tantra!

When you're a Tantra practitioner, you're creating love, and as those sages The Beatles remind us, "Love is all you need."

You're actively feeding your health and happiness and possibly warding off aging and dementia.

If you're in a committed relationship, you're constantly renewing what you've got. There's nothing like ecstatic connecting to keep the home fires burning bright. Tantra relationships have an anti-staleness factor built into them.

If you're not in a committed relationship, it's about as fun a way to be single as you can find. I don't know about you, but I'd much rather spend hours practicing Tantra than refining my golf stroke.

And did I mention that the sex is amazing?

SEXY SUMMARY

TANTRA IS OFTEN misrepresented and misunderstood.

THE GOAL OF 'RED TANTRA' is to achieve union with the Beloved within. This is done in erotic partnership with another person. Tantra unifies the partners' energies so that the sum of their energy is greater than its parts, a sort of energetic big bang results, and it takes them to a place of transcendent bliss.

AMONG THE THINGS TANTRA STUDENTS LEARN are how to locate and move energy, activate the chakras, quiet the mind, expand their orgasm, do sacred-spot massage, integrate stillness into their lovemaking, and practice specific foreplay and intercourse techniques.

TANTRA IS A WONDERFUL WAY to dazzle your dates, keep yourself and your relationship healthy, and have amazing sex.

Sex and relationship expert **REID MIHALKO** *of ReidAboutSex.com is the creator and founder of Relationship10x.com and Sex10xOnline.com, as well as the world-famous CuddleParty.com and SexGeekSummerCamp.com.*

Reid helps adults create more self-esteem, self-confidence and greater health in their relationships and sex lives using an inspiring mixture of humor and knowledge.

Reid's workshops, online courses, live events, and college lectures have been attended by over 50,000 men and women. He has appeared in media such as Oprah's Our America With Lisa Ling on OWN, the Emmy award-winning talk show Montel, Dr. Phil's The Doctors on CBS, Bravo's Miss Advised, Fox News, in Newsweek, Seventeen, GQ, The Washington Post, and in thirteen countries and at least seven languages.

You can contact Reid at Reid@ReidAboutSex.com, follow him on Twitter via http://Twitter.com/ReidAboutSex and on FB via http://Facebook.com/ReidAboutSex

CHAPTER SEVENTEEN

Energy Sex

by Reid Mihalko & Carl Frankel

A MAN WHO HAS NO USE OF HIS GENITALS OR LOWER BODY, WHO has no sensation from the ribcage down and very little dexterity in his hands, has a thriving sex life and regularly makes women scream with pleasure.

A woman who finds orgasms from vaginal penetration challenging has 'eargasms' complete with multiple orgasms and squirting when a friend puts his fingers in her ears.

Unbelievable though these stories sound, they're true. I know because the quadriplegic gentleman is a colleague of mine who's shown me firsthand what he can do, and the 'eargasm' woman's friend is, that's right, me.

How are Jedi-like sexual feats such as these possible?

Through energy sex, the topic of this chapter.

The Joy of (Energy) Sex

Energy sex is what happens when we engage and play with sensual and erotic energy. Energy sex can be done solo, with a partner, or in groups. It doesn't depend on gender or anatomy. It doesn't require an erect penis or accessible vulva, nor does it care whether you're gay or straight, a virgin or a player. If you and your partners are skilled enough, you don't even have to be in the same room together. It's actually been done over Skype!

There's nothing special about the many people who consciously play with sexual energy. Anyone can do it—it's a learnable skill. If my quadriplegic friend can learn to run energy, so can you, so long as you've got an open mind and are willing to put in the time and effort.

Energy sex is a winner for many reasons, starting with the fact that it enhances your erotic repertoire and provides an alternative pathway for giving and receiving enormous pleasure. You know that box of four crayons you get at the Italian restaurant for doodling on the paper tablecloth? That's what our mainstream culture gives us sexually. We don't even get the box of eight crayons we got in kindergarten, never mind the full set of 64 crayons that's available! Having a bigger box of crayons to play with makes sex more interesting, and when you make sex more interesting, you make life more interesting. Energy sex gives us access to all the colors and bandwidths that are our erotic birthright.

Energy sex can also be a way to have safe sex—not "safer sex," but totally safe, no-body-parts-touching-your-partner sex. (You can combine energy sex with hands-on, parts-in sex, but it's entirely optional.)

Energy sex can also be an emotionally safer way to have sex. With penetrative 'sex-sex,' it's easy for people to get energetically and emotionally entangled. There's premature ejaculation, and there's also premature attachment. Jack or Jill has a one-night stand and falls in love; they start creating fantasies about building a life with the other person before it makes sense to do so. We're all acquainted with examples of this; we may have done it ourselves. Premature attachment can also happen with energy sex, but because there's less physical entanglement it's less likely.*

Finally, energy sex is magical in the sense that it's not easily explained by our rational mind. It feels improbable and miraculous, even for those of us who've run energy many times. It's literally a wonderful experience, as in—full of wonder. The world becomes wondrous and fresh as it was when we were children. I don't know anyone who wouldn't benefit from more magic in their life.

The Energy Sex Experience

People experience sexual energy differently. Some people get twitchy as the energy moves through them. The word for this, which comes to us from the kundalini yoga tradition, is *kriya*. Others show no visible changes but 'feel' something happening, while some people show no change and feel nothing happening—but the people they play with feel all sorts of things!

Because everyone experiences sexual energy differently, I find it works best to describe energy sex by analogy. Imagine flying a kite. From the ground, you can't tell how hard the wind is blowing up where the kite is. The wind is basically invisible, but we feel its effect in our bodies through the kite string.

---

* It *is* a risk, though, which is why I recommend using visualization rituals to ensure that the partners' energies remain healthily independent when the energy sex is over. Healthy, ongoing emotional and energetic connections require the participants to consciously exercise autonomy. Otherwise, the unconscious impulse to merge and entangle can get in the way.

With practice, we can learn to work with, rather than fight, the wind by letting string out or taking it in, or by shifting our location on the ground. We maneuver the kite by learning how to be in relationship with the wind.

Playing with sexual energy is like playing with the wind. You can't see it, but you can sense and play with it. And, like our kite-flier, you can learn to control and harness it. You can reel sexual energy in or let it soar. Once you become skilled enough, your kite can even become one of those stunt kites with two sets of strings. Now you can do the energy-sex equivalent of dives, loops and tricks with your body's energy and your lover's. What a fun way to play!

Here's what energy sex boils down to: You experience energy as real and as something you can exercise control or influence over—and then you play with it erotically.

If you're having partnered sex, the energy can show up like a separate presence. Two separate presences, really, because there's my energy and your energy—and if you want to get really geeky, there are also our physical bodies and the frequency of our energy combined, making five 'presences' in all. Together they're like musical instruments contributing to the making of a song. Practice enough and you'll be like the orchestra's conductor. A co-conductor, really, because the person you're playing with will be orchestrating the music, too.

And, as we've seen, physical touching isn't required.

How about physical responses? Does arousal happen? How about orgasms? Yes to physical arousal. Men often (but not always) get an erection, or have erections phase in and out. Women also get turned on, with or without lubrication (which is the case for sex-sex, too). In fact, many women say energy sex is as good for them (or better than) penetrative sex!

As for orgasms, that depends on how you define the term. What we usually think of as an orgasm is a physical event characterized by intense, involuntary, muscular contractions in the genitals and pelvis, usually with pleasurable sensations and the release of muscular tension. For men, these are usually wet orgasms—they ejaculate semen. Most women don't ejaculate when they have physical orgasms, although some do.

And then there are energy orgasms. These are pleasurable in much the same way as physical orgasms, but they aren't centered in the genitals. They're experienced as involuntary waves of pleasure that sweep over the whole body, or as pleasurable spikes or peaks of sensation that are centered in one or more areas of the body. Those *kriyas* I mentioned earlier? They're the energy-sex equivalent of a standard orgasm's muscle spasm in the pelvis. Energy orgasm *kriyas* can be mini-ones, like a twitchy leg, a ringing in the ears, or even a spontaneous giggle fit. Energy orgasms can last seconds or go on for hours. They can also look like huge bursts of body-shaking energy that whip your head back, cause you to cry out, or even inspire you to go into yoga poses (which has happened to me). They can also be experienced genitally and feel similar to your standard orgasm.

No one type of *kriya* is "better" or more evolved than another. And, as we've said, some people don't experience kriyas every time or experience them at all. Everyone is different and everyone is perfect.

When energy sex without physical touching produces orgasms, they're usually energy orgasms. Full-on physical orgasms can occur, but they're more rare.*

If you're rolling your eyes at all this orgasm-without-touching talk, I can relate—I have a healthy Inner Skeptic, too. And yet history is full of miraculous-seeming things that have rational explanations. When electricity and light bulbs were first introduced, imagine how people reacted when they flipped a switch and light came on in the darkness of night! It was simultaneously impossible and happening—a miracle that had an explanation. Maybe the time will come when we understand the science of erotic energy better and energy sex becomes something we take for granted, like electricity.

Just because our skeptical mind tells us something isn't possible doesn't make it so. We need to be skeptical about our skepticism, too, and allow ourselves to explore the unknown without closing off to it.

Is Energy Sex 'Sex?'

This is a reasonable question if you're among the many people who believe sex has to include physically touching your partner.

My answer is yes, definitely. For one thing, it involves the co-creation of pleasurable erotic sensations and that's a plausible definition of sexual activity even if physically touching another person isn't involved. For another, it aligns with our consensus understanding of what sex means. If Janet was in a monogamous relationship with Chris and reported that she'd had energy sex with their neighbor, but not to worry because they hadn't actually touched each other, how do you think Chris would react? Especially if Janet reported that her *kriyas* triggered squirting orgasms as well: "But, darling, he never touched me!"

*** It can be difficult to distinguish between the two, especially if you're a vulva-owning woman or F-to-M (Female-to-Male) Trans-Man.**

If something delivers pleasure like sex and triggers jealousy like sex, it probably is sex. And even if energy sex isn't sex to you, it's better to negotiate as if it is.

Resonance Play

As a teacher, I find that what I call *Resonance Play* is the best way to learn to play with sexual energy.

A simple science experiment that's done in grade-school classrooms around the world illustrates the foundational principle of Resonance Play. Take two tuning forks of the same exact note. Connect Tuning Fork A to some basic electronic measuring equipment that measures slight vibrations. Take Tuning Fork B and walk it across the room (or even across the length of a football field) and strike it so it starts vibrating. When the sound waves that come off Tuning Fork B reach Tuning Fork A, Tuning Fork A will begin vibrating. All hail science!

If we hooked Tuning Fork B up to a device that allowed us to increase the strength of its vibrations, we'd see that Tuning Fork A would begin to vibrate more forcefully along with B. If I were to keep increasing the volume on Tuning Fork B, there would come a time when Tuning Fork A's vibrations began affecting Tuning Fork B, too, creating a feedback loop between the two tuning forks that tremendously magnifies the vibratory energy between the two.

The basic concept of Resonance Play is this: We're all walking tuning forks. You learn to tune your note like you might tune a guitar string to match your partner's 'note.' Then you increase the volume on your note to start your partner vibrating like Tuning Fork A. You continue to increase your volume until your partner's vibrations start making you vibrate more. Soon enough, the feedback loop effect kicks in and the sexual energy magnifies tremendously, at which point, if all goes well, you've got enough energy (or 'wind' if we go back to the kite analogy) to stunt fly your kites!

How Does Energy Speak To You?

Before you can match your energy with someone else's, you'll first want to know how energy speaks to you.

Here's a real-world example most people can relate to that will help you decipher how energy shows up for you. Let's say you're hanging out with some friends and someone really angry walks into the room. Do you notice how the energy in the room shifts when that happens? Now take a moment and ask yourself how you experience the shift. Some people feel it in their gut. For others, it's auditory—the room somehow sounds different. For some, the shift might be visual, with everything from the colors in the room becoming brighter or more dull, to the air itself seeming to vibrate or seem full of moving, translucent balls or bubbles of color. And for yet others, a shift in energy isn't associated with any of the five physical senses, but experienced as a vague 'something' on the periphery of their awareness.

It's the same with erotic energy. Some people hear it, others see it, and some feel it in their bodies. I've even met people who taste it. Energy also speaks to some people in the form of ideas or visuals in their mind's eye. For others, the experience comes to them through the emotions—it's an empathetic experience.

We're all wired differently and no one way of experiencing energy is better or worse than another. Your way is just that—your way.

Regardless of how energy speaks to you, it's always an inner awareness, a special type of intention, that allows us to connect to energy. Always. You can't 'left brain' think your way into tuning into energy and you can't force it, either. Your relationship with energy is already present, just like the sound of your heartbeat is happening as you read this, but it's usually too subtle for you to be aware of it. If, like most of us, you have trouble accessing inner awareness of your energies, that's usually because there's too much noise—too much stress and too many thoughts—in the way. Or because you lack the knowhow, practice and experience. Or, that's right, both!

Whatever the blocks, the good news is that thousands if not millions of people have learned to have energy sex. And so can you.

It's About Awareness, It's About Attitude

Playing with sexual energy requires you to pick up signals at a very subtle level. It may not look fine-grained when people are having explosive *kriyas* or screaming in the throes of ecstasy, but all that energy comes from a nuanced place. It's as if you're playing an electric guitar: Small, intentional moves are amplified into large experiences.

Tuning into energy at this subtle level requires a special type of awareness that requires your parasympathetic nervous system to be engaged. To explain: We have two parallel nervous systems in our bodies. The sympathetic nervous system is activated by stress: it triggers our fight-or-flight response. The parasympathetic nervous system kicks in when we don't feel at risk and it feels safe to relax. A lot of us are constantly stressed out and have difficulty accessing the parasympathetic nervous system's relaxation response. This is a problem at both the individual and broader societal levels. When people forget how to relax, their blood pressure goes up, the incidence of heart attacks increases, and they are more prone to a host of other medical problems, too.

Being stressed out also intrudes on people's ability not only to have energy sex, but to have sex-sex, too. You can't orgasm when you're being chased by a bear—and you can't energy-orgasm, either, or for that matter tune into the subtle levels at which energy is contacted and played with. It's really difficult to run energy if you don't drop all that stress and noise so you can 'go parasympathetic' and tune into the subtle energetic levels.

That's right: Every time you do energy sex, you're taking a vacation from fight-and-flight. Not only is it good for your blood pressure and health, it's like lying on a Hawaiian beach—with orgasms!

In addition to going parasympathetic, you also have to believe that energy sex is possible. Or, at a minimum, you need to suspend disbelief. Attitude matters with energy sex. A lot. The more you're ready to believe in it, the greater the chances are that you'll experience it as real and have a great energy-sex experience.

Every time you do energy sex, you're taking a vacation from fight-and-flight.

But is energy sex real? As in, 'really real?' I'll have more to say about that shortly. For now, I'll simply note that at the end of the day, I don't really care if energy sex is 'really real.' I want to have fun and enjoy great connections with others. If you and I do that via a shared delusion, so what? What matters to me is that the pleasure is real; the joy is real; the connection is real. If energy sex helps me explore and connect and have fun with others and myself, three cheers for energy sex!

When you practice energy sex, you're training at being open-minded in two distinct senses of the term—receptive, and free (as much as possible) of limiting preconceptions. The more you can be open-minded in this double sense, the more intimate and pleasurable your experience will be for both you and your partner.

If your partner can do the same, the odds go way up that you'll get into a great parasympathetic Resonance Play groove together. You'll feed off each other and eventually what psychologists call a confidence/competence loop will kick in, with "Yes, I can!" feeding "Yes, I'm good at this!" in a spiral that increases everyone's pleasure.

Here's another side benefit of energy sex: It's a training ground for great habits and can make you more self-confident and open-minded. Energy sex has made me a happier, better person and it can do the same for you.

Ya Gotta Believe

You won't be able to experience the pleasures of energy sex if your Inner Skeptic keeps getting in the way. Here are three rational arguments to chill out that voice in your head.

First: Scientists are beginning to explain the energy sex experience. The data aren't conclusive yet, but they're suggestive and intriguing. The basic notion is this: Babies are herky-jerky in their motions. They learn over time to be less so. They do this by learning to regulate their neuromuscular system. Let's say I want to touch my nose with my finger. As an infant, I initially smack myself in the face with my whole hand. Then I start to get the hang of it until I can eventually make a smooth movement with my index finger landing gently on target. I do this by firing certain muscle fibers and keeping other ones from moving (the technical word is 'inhibiting'). From that point on, it happens automatically. Once we're past the infant stage, we don't have to pay attention to touching our nose, we just do it.

As we've seen, *kriyas* are the twitchy motions some people make when erotic energy is moving through them. Some scientists and brain geeks believe that these *kriyas* are the visible manifestation of what happens when nervous pathways that were previously inhibited become *disinhibited*. It's as if, in this limited sense, we become babies again—we're less in control of the energy moving through us and so we move in an uncontrolled, herky-jerky way.

> *We need to be skeptical about our skepticism, too.*

If the scientists are right about this—and they're using brain scan machines to study this—then the energy we play with during energy sex is as real as the energy we use to scratch our nose. Only it's disinhibited energy, energy we don't control via our usual neuromuscular control mechanisms.

With practice, you can learn how to consciously turn your inhibitor switch on or off depending on the situation. You can 'go energetic' when the time is right and you can be 'normal' when that's what's called for. You probably don't want to be shaking uncontrollably when you're dining with the President. Or your future in-laws.

So that's the first bullet point in my Skeptic Reassurance Program: Scientists are coming up with a plausible explanation for the energy part of energy sex. (They already knew about the sex part.)

Here's my second way to soothe the skeptical beast: The innumerable anecdotal accounts of people who've played with energy erotically and reported similar experiences. This evidence goes back millennia. Not only do we have the Tantric and Taoist sexuality traditions with their ancient texts, pictures and statuary, but we can also view ecstatic religious behaviors such as speaking in tongues and the quaking that gave Quakers their name as variations on the kriyatic experience. Are all the past and current practitioners of energy sex in all its forms and traditions lying? No, and we're probably not deluded, either. (Not all of us, anyway.)

Here's my third and final point to help you cognitively merge science and mysticism. Let's say you haven't been persuaded by the emerging scientific explanation for kriyas or by the anecdotal evidence. Let's also say everybody who's ever had energy sex has been making it up. The experience can still be experienced as real due to the scientifically proven placebo effect. It's the old story of mind over matter: If someone with a disease is given a sugar pill and told it contains an ingredient that will make them better, a significant percentage of patients will show progress because they believe they'll get better.

In addition, people have mirror neurons that help us pick up on and experience other people's feelings. This means that if you're experiencing energy running through you, even if it's a delusion, I may feel the same thing, too. We create and can share in each other's reality.

If both partners believe that energy sex is real, they can co-create and enjoy the benefits of an energy sex experience. From a pragmatist's perspective, so what if it's a shared delusion so long as it's consensual and everyone's having fun? The feel-good hormones and endorphins released are real.

Your Lover Is a Wineglass

Have you ever tried to make a wineglass sing? If you have, you'll know that four things are involved. There's speed or rate—how fast you move your finger around the glass. There's pressure—how hard or soft you touch the glass. There's friction—how wet or dry your finger (or the glass) needs to be. These are the three physical things you need to pay attention to. And the fourth requirement? It's where your attention goes—more specifically, how you adjust your attention so that you find that place in your awareness where you can make the wineglass sing.

As you relax into varying the speed, pressure and friction and move closer to making the wine glass sing, where does your attention go? Who do you 'become?' Do you 'listen' to the wineglass with your fingertip? Do you 'tune in' with your gut? Is your 'wineglass place' a few inches inside your ear? What happens to your eyes? Do they take in the entire wineglass with a soft focus or is your gaze sharply focused on one specific point? Do you close your eyes?

When you've made the right adjustments to your perceptual and nervous system so you can sense whether you're getting closer to making the glass hum or moving further away, that's what I call your 'wineglass place.' When you're having energy sex, this is where you want to go when you tune into your lover.*

Your wineglass place is like a Spider-Man sixth sense. It's where you'll best be able to tune into someone else's frequency so you can have great energy sex with them.

Playing with Sexual Energy

If you want to have energy sex, you'll first need to get in touch with your own energy. While anyone can do this, it's easier for some than others. It helps to have an activity that involves body awareness. Hobbies like ecstatic dance, tango, contact improv, massage, tai chi, chi gong and yoga can help you become more embodied.

You can also take a class on an esoteric erotic tradition or energy sex. While you usually won't find this sort of thing at your local community college, there are good teachers out there. The more information and support you get, the easier it will be to become proficient at energy sex.

You don't need a partner to play with energy—you can also do it during solo sex time. I recommend this highly, and not only because it's fun. Solo play is when you hone your ability to engage with others energetically. Imagine a basketball ace who's mastered the ability to make the basketball do their bidding. They make their teammates better. The same is true in the bedroom. Those hours spent dribbling and shooting on the court are what make you a great person to play with. (Double entendres intended.)

What the Taoists call the Microcosmic Orbit is a great way to become energy-sensitive. This is covered in Michael Winn's chapter on non-ejaculatory male orgasm, so I won't discuss it at length here. Suffice it to say that I highly recommend it for learning how to build and move energy, alone or with a partner.

Other ways to build sexual energy are breath, sound, and pelvic floor work. On their own they're effective, and combined they're all the more so:

- Breath. You can inhale through your nose and out through your mouth, or vice-versa. If you're playing with a partner, you can inhale and exhale together, or alternatively one of you inhales while the other exhales. Make

* This also applies to when you're having sex-sex.

sure you breathe deeply and use your diaphragm! If you breathe too fast, you can reduce the amount of carbon dioxide in your bloodstream. This can cause you to feel buzzy and make it next to impossible to pick up on the subtle sensations of sensual energy, especially if you're a beginner.

- Sound. When you release a long stream of sound, especially the kind of sound that vibrates your chest so that you can feel it in your hand when you put your hand over your breast bone, you activate the vagus nerve, which runs from your brain down into your pelvis. This, in turn, activates your parasympathetic nervous system, which as we've seen makes it easier to tune into sexual energy. If you want to further stimulate your vagus nerve, stick your tongue out like a Kali the Destroyer statue during your sound exhale. Yup, sticking out your tongue and saying 'Aaah' will help you have better energy sex!
- Pelvic Floor Work. You can build sexual energy by squeezing and releasing your pelvic floor muscles—pubococcygeus or 'PC' muscles—with what is commonly known as Kegel exercises or Kegels. Feel free to experiment with different patterns. You can contract your PC muscles while you inhale or while you exhale. You can pump them fast or slow, hold them for a few seconds or not. Explore. Play. Investigate.

If you're with a partner, you can do these exercises with your eyes closed or while eye-gazing. Both have their place, but I especially recommend eye-gazing. It's a great way to connect, and some emerging research suggests that eye-gazing and being in close proximity to another person's welcoming facial expression may trigger parasympathetic nervous system activity. Are you seeing a pattern here?

I'm also a big fan of visualization. My personal experience suggests that the act of imagining energy moving accelerates actual physical activity. We'll know soon enough if this is true: A prominent research doctor and I are testing whether visualizing energy moving up and down one's spine increases electrical activity in that area. If it does—and I'm betting the answer will be 'yes'—then that would make visualization techniques combined with switching off your inhibitor switch and dropping into your parasympathetic nervous system the Big Three of energy sex.

Keeping It Real

We're all human. Things rarely, if ever, go perfectly. You can pretty much count on having stumbles when you're running energy. Even after you've gotten to the wineglass place, there'll be times when you lose that connection.

You may fall out of synch with your partner. The phone may ring. Your Inner Skeptic may start squawking.

If you lose your focus, take a breath, let out some sound, and re-group. Share with your partner what's happening so you stay connected with them. Remind yourself that losing the thread and then finding it again is just part of the game. Things won't always go perfectly, and who cares? The important thing is that you're playing, learning and connecting.

Reality is bigger and more wondrous than any of us can imagine. Energy sex offers a wonderful way to explore the reality that lies beyond our narrow Italian restaurant, four crayon-set confines. It's a way to open to the Mystery that lies beyond the reach of our narrow, rational minds. A way to say yes. A way to grow.

And: You can reap tremendous rewards from energy sex without having a spiritual bone in your body. It's a great way to enhance regular 'sex-sex' and on its own it's also a wonderful way to play. At the end of the day, the most compelling rationale may be this one—energy sex is good, clean, fabulous fun.

SEXY SUMMARY

ENERGY SEX IS A FUN, rewarding way to play erotically that anyone can learn.

IT'S A WAY TO PRACTICE TOTALLY SAFE SEX because you don't need to touch your partner.

ENERGY SEX is a bit like flying a kite. You can't see the wind, but you can sense it and play with it.

THE FIRST THING TO DO is learn how you experience energy yourself.

TO PLAY WITH YOUR PARTNER'S ENERGY, you'll want to go to the 'wineglass place.'

THE THREE KEYS TO ENERGY SEX appear to be visualization, relaxing (going into your parasympathetic nervous system) and switching off your neuromuscular 'inhibitor switch.'

Resources

The Dance of Anatomy and Energy (Sheri Winston)

BOOKS

Atlas of Human Anatomy (Frank H. Netter)

Intimate Communion: Awakening Your Sexual Essence (David Deida)

New View of A Woman's Body (Federation of Feminist Women's Health Centers)

Passion Play (Felice Dunas)

Succulent SexCraft: Your Hands-On Guide to Erotic Play & Practice (Sheri Winston with Carl Frankel)

The Clitoral Truth (Rebecca Chalker)

Women's Anatomy of Arousal: Secret Maps to Buried Pleasure (Sheri Winston)

ONLINE CLASSES

Secrets of Female Pleasure: Women's Anatomy of Arousal (http://intimateartscenter.com/shop/downloadwebinars)

Oral Sex (Carlyle Jansen)

DVD's

Going Down: The Official Guide (Good Releasing)

Head's Up: The Official Guide (Good Releasing)

Oral Sex For Couples (Jaiya/New World Sex Education)

Tristan Taormino's Expert Guide to Cunnilingus (Vivid)

Tristan Taormino's Expert Guide to Fellatio (Vivid)

BOOKS

Blow Each Other Away (Jaiya)

Blow Him Away: How to Give Him Mind-Blowing Oral Sex (Marcy Michaels)

Hot Sex Tips, Tricks and Licks (Jessica O'Reilly)

How to Be a Great Lover (Lou Paget)

How to Give Her Absolute Pleasure (Lou Paget)

She Comes First (Ian Kerner)

The Lowdown on Going Down (Marcy Michaels)

The Oral Sex Deck: 50 His & Her Tongue Techniques for Toe-Curling Ecstasy (Beverly Cummings)

Tickle His Pickle (Sadie Allison)

Ultimate Guide to Cunnilingus (Violet Blue)

Ultimate Guide to Fellatio (Violet Blue)

Anal Sex (Jon Pressick)

BOOKS

Anal Pleasure and Health: A Guide for Men Women and Couples (Jack Morin)

Baby Got Back: Anal Erotica (edited by Rachel Kramer Bussel)

The Ultimate Guide to Anal Sex for Men (Tristan Taormino)

The Ultimate Guide to Anal Sex for Women (Tristan Taormino)

The Ultimate Guide to Prostate Pleasure: Erotic Explorations for Men and Their Partners (Charlie Glickman and Aislinn Emirzian)

VIDEO

Tristan Taormino's Expert Guide to Advanced Anal Sex

Tristan Taormino's Expert Guide to Advanced Anal Sex for Men

Power Exchange (Nina Hartley & Ernest Greene)

Back on the Ropes (Two Knotty Boys)

Becoming a Slave (Jack Rinella)

Bondage for Sex (Chanta Rose((no Kindle)

Come Hither: A Commonsense Guide To Kinky Sex (Gloria G. Brame)

Consensual Sadomasochism: How To Talk About It and Do It Safely (William A. Henkin & Sybil Holliday)

Erotic Bondage Handbook (Jay Wiseman)

Erotic Slavehood: A Miss Abernathy Omnibus (Christina Abernathy)

Flogging (Joseph Bean)

Partners in Power (Jack Rinella)

Screw the Roses, Send Me the Thorns (Philip Miller & Molly Devon)

Sensuous Magic (Pat Califia)

Shibari You Can Use: Japanese Rope Bondage (Lee Bridgett Harrington) (no Kindle)

SM 101 (Jay Wiseman)

The Loving Dominant (John Warren)

The Mistress Manual: The Good Girl's Guide to Female Dominance (Mistress Lorelei)

The New Bottoming Book (Janet W. Hardy & Dossie Easton)

The New Topping Book (Janet Hardy & Dossie Easton)

The Sexually Dominant Woman: A Workbook for Nervous Beginners (Lady Green)

Toybag Guide to Canes and Caning (Janet Hardy)

Two Knotty Boys Showing You The Ropes: A Step-by-Step, Illustrated Guide for Tying Sensual and Decorative Rope Bondage

Touch (Joseph Kramer)

Red-Hot Touch: A Head-to-Toe Handbook for Mind-Blowing Orgasms (Jaiya & Jon Hanauer)

The New School of Erotic Touch (www.eroticmassage.com)

Finding the Lover Within (Caroline Muir)

The Sexual Healing Journey: A Guide for Survivors of Sexual Abuse, 3rd Edition (Wendy Maltz)

Healing Sex: A Mind-Body Approach to Healing Sexual Trauma (Staci Haines)

Sexual Healing: The Tantra Way (Charles Muir)

Sex as Improv and Creative Play (Karen B.K. Chan)

BOOKS

Brown, Stuart. 2009. *Play: How It Shapes the Brain, Opens the Imagination, and Invigorates the Soul* (Avery)

Johnstone, Keith. 1987. *Impro: Improvisation and the Theatre* (Routledge)

Millar, Thomas MacAulay. 2008. "Toward a Performance Model of Sex", in *Yes Means Yes: Visions of Female Sexual Power and A World Without Rape* (Eds. Jaclyn Friedman and Jessica Valenti). Seal Press.

Morin, Jack. 1989. *The Erotic Mind: Unlocking the Inner Sources of Passion and Fulfillment (*Harper Perennial)

Zaporah, Ruth. 1995. *Action Theatre: The Improvisation of Presence (*North Atlantic Books)

ONLINE CLASSES

Chan, Karen B. K. 2013. "Jam", a 5-minute animation on having improvisational sex. http://www.fluidexchange.org

Sex and Shame (Charlie Glickman)

Blog of anonymous stories about sex and sexuality (dotellstories.tumblr.com/)

Keeping the Flame Alive (Jessica O'Reilly & Nadine Thornhill)

Passionate Marriage: Keeping Love and Intimacy Alive in Committed Relationships (David Schnarch)

Rekindling Desire *(Barry and Emily McCarthy)*

Sexual Intelligence: What We Really Want from Sex—and How to Get It (Marty Klein)

Fantasy, Role Play and Communication (Megan Andelloux)

Hot and Fast (Megan Andelloux)

A Billion Wicked Thoughts: What the Internet Tells Us About Sexual Relationships (Ogi Ogas and Sai Gaddam)

Taking Sides, Clashing Views in Abnormal Psychology (Richard Halgin, 6th ed.)

Extended Female Orgasm (Patti Taylor)

Available at ExpandedLovemaking.com

Expand Her Orgasm Tonight

The Seduction Trilogy

Also, links to Taylor's podcasts on Personal Life Media, The Expanded Lovemaking Show

On Amazon.com

Expanded Orgasm, Second Edition (Patricia Taylor, book)

Expand Her Orgasm Tonight (Patricia Taylor, DVD)

Non-Ejaculatory Male Orgasm (Michael Winn)

DVD AND AUDIO CD COURSES

Sexual Vitality Qigong DVD (Michael Winn)

Healing Love: Taoist Sexual Secrets (Michael Winn & Joyce Gayheart)

Medical & Spiritual Qigong Fundamentals 1 & 2 (Michael Winn)

Emotional Alchemy: Fusion of 5 Elements 1, 2, 3 (Michael Winn)

BOOKS AND E-BOOKS

Way of the Inner Smile: Tao Path to Peace & Self-Acceptance

Taoist Secrets of Love: Cultivating Male Sexual Energy (Michael Winn & Mantak Chia)

Healing Love Through the Tao: Cultivating Female Sexual Energy (Mantak & Maneewan Chia, ghostwritten by Michael Winn)

ARTICLES AND FAQS

Quest for Spiritual Orgasm: Taoist and Tantric Sexual Practices in the West

Transforming Sexual Energy with Water-and-Fire Alchemy

FAQs on Taoist Sexual Practices

Sexual Qigong and Sexual Identity: Tao Cosmology Talk

The Tao of Cultivating Sexual Energy

OTHER

China Dream Trip (for spiritual adventurers who want to cultivate themselves in Taoist sacred mountains of China.

These resources can be found at HealingTaoUSA.com.

Female Ejaculation (Tallulah Sulis)

BOOKS

Female Ejaculation and the G Spot (Deborah Sundahl)
Heart Of The Flower (Andrew Barnes)
The Multi-Orgasmic Couple (Mantak Chia)

DVD's

Annie Sprinkle's Herstory of Porn
Divine Nectar: A Guide to Female Ejaculation
G Spot Wisdom
Healing Sex
Liquid Love
Magic Gold

ONLINE INFO PRODUCTS

FemaleLiquidOrgasm.com
MakeAnyWomanSquirt.com
SquirtYourHeartOut.com
Intimate ArtsCenter.com. Online class (Sheri Winston): The Fountain of the Goddess: The Learnable Art of Female Ejaculation

Bondassage (Jaeleen Bennis)

Bondassage: Kinky Erotic Massage Tips For Lovers (Jaeleen Bennis and Eve Minax)

Tantra (Charles Muir)

BOOKS

Tantra: The Art of Conscious Loving (Charles Muir & Caroline Muir)

DVDS, CDS & MULTI-MEDIA

Secrets of Female Sexual Ecstasy (Charles Muir & Caroline Muir)
Meeting of The Masters, Vol. 1: Alchemy, Orgasm and Awakening
Meeting of The Masters, Vol. 2: Sex, Energy and Ecstatic Love
Meeting of The Masters, Vol. 3: Eastern Secrets of Sexual Love (Charles Muir and Mantak Chia)
The Sacred Spot: A Complete Guide to Female Sexual Awakening (Charles Muir)
Holy Relationship (Charles Muir)
White Tantra Instruction (Charles Muir)

For more information: SourceTantra.com

Energy Sex (Reid Mihalko)

Urban Tantra: Sacred Sex for the Twenty-First Century (Barbara Carrellas)
Energetic Play workshops with Monique Darling (DivineInterludes.com)